Natural Bodycare

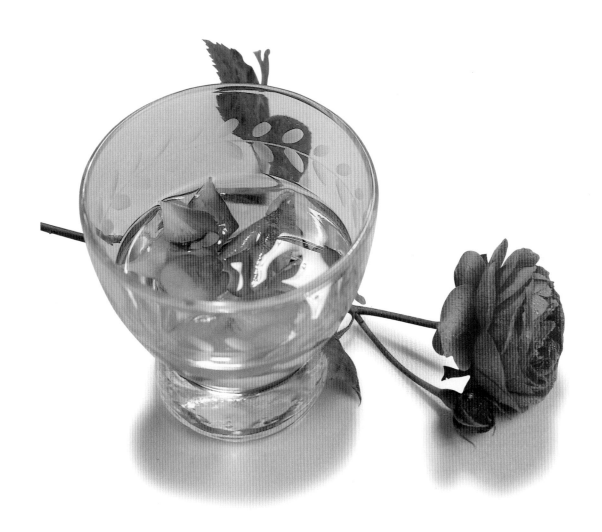

Natural Bodycare

Creating Aromatherapy Cosmetics
for Health & Beauty

Julia Meadows
photography by Wm B. Dewey

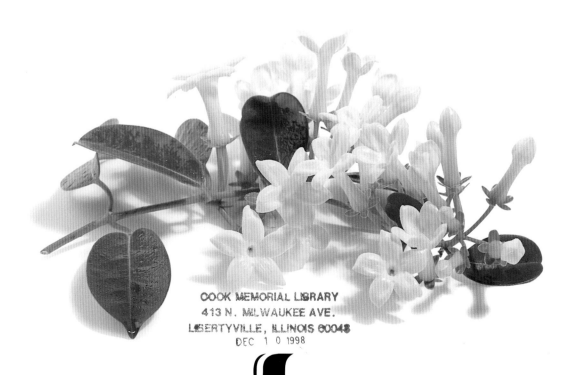

Sterling Publishing Co., Inc. New York

Natural Bodycare:
Creating Aromatherapy Cosmetics for Health and Beauty
is dedicated to my husband, Orville

Library of Congress Cataloging-in-Publication Data Available

10 9 8 7 6 5 4 3 2 1

Published by Sterling Publishing Company, Inc.
387 Park Avenue South, New York, N.Y. 10016

© 1998 by Julia Meadows

Distributed in Canada by Sterling Publishing,
c/o Canadian Manda Group, One Atlantic Avenue, Suite 105, Toronto, Ontario, Canada M6K 3E7

Distributed in Great Britain and Europe by Cassell PLC,
Wellington House, 125 Strand, London, England WC2R 0BB

Distributed in Australia by Capricorn Link (Australia) Pty Ltd.,
P.O. Box 6651, Baulkham Hills Business Centre, NSW, Australia 2153

The projects in this book are the original creations of the author. They may be reproduced by individuals for personal pleasure; reproduction on a larger scale with the intent of personal profit is prohibited.

Every effort has been made to ensure that all the information in this book is accurate. However, due to differing conditions, tools, and individual skills, the author and publisher assume no responsibility or liability for any injuries, losses or other damages that may result, directly or indirectly, from the use of essential oils and aromatherapy formulas or any information contained in this book.

Printed in Hong Kong

ISBN 0-8069-4245-2

Contents

Preface

I am often asked how I got involved in the innovative and unusual field of natural bodycare and true aromatherapy. My personal epiphany came in 1986, and, as it does for many people, it resulted from a deep desire to make life changes, accompanied by a series of 'messages' that seemed to signal that change was inevitable. For years, I had followed a rewarding career practicing corporate architecture and design, but as time went on, the high stress and demanding nature of the work began to take an unseen toll. I had moved to California in search of something more, wanting to combine my creative career with personal development. Little did I guess what I would find once I arrived!

Growing up in the English countryside, I had been raised in natural surroundings and learned a great deal about plants, herbs and natural remedies from my parents. During my early career years, though, I totally ignored everything I knew about natural living and allowed myself to be caught up in the frenzied search for success and achievement. Everything 'natural' seemed quaintly old-fashioned in the sophisticated, high-tech late 1970's and early 1980's. This continued until I reached Los Angeles, my dream of so many years, where a health crisis threatened to cut short everything I had worked towards. All of a sudden, I found I was reacting strangely to everyday substances — cosmetics, household cleaners, medicines, even certain foods! One of my most enjoyable pastimes, searching department stores for the newest perfumes and body products, inevitably resulted in uncontrollable sneezing, teary eyes and severe headaches. Skin products itched and burned and produced bizarre rashes and sensitivities. My energy level dropped, and I felt inexplicably overwhelmed and exhausted most of the time. Medical analysis turned up nothing concrete, but my quality of life was so compromised that I was determined to get to the root of the problem and solve the mystery.

It took some time, but I came to discover what many other people are also currently experiencing. The human organism is a miraculous entity, but when personal and professional pressures are just too much, most of us are not fully aware of the stress we have put ourselves under until our health suffers in some way. We are then given messages to make changes and seek a more balanced way of living. I determined to make changes in my lifestyle, career, relationships, diet and outlook,

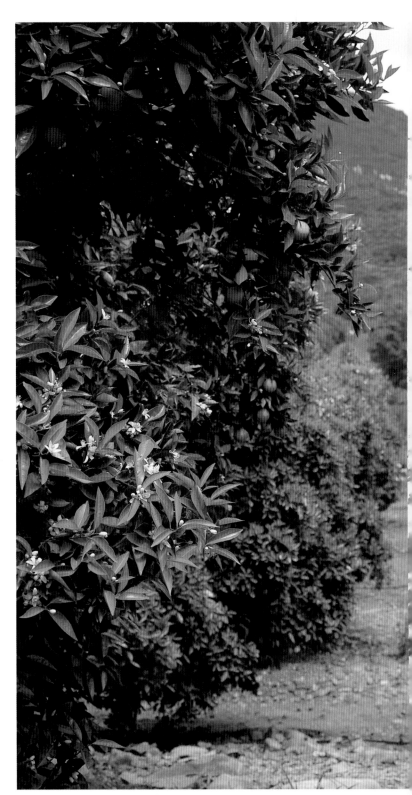

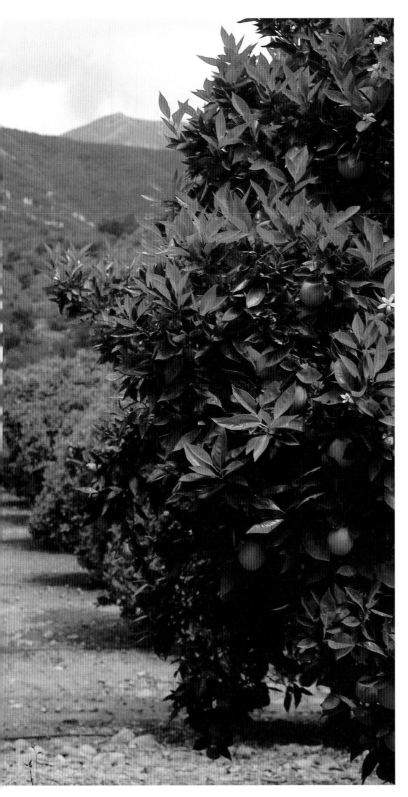

and decided to re-examine what I knew about alternate modalities and natural remedies. Along the way, I was fortunate to discover aromatherapy. This ancient art and science is a fundamentally a branch of herbalism and offers us the benefits of this natural therapy in an immediate and potent way. The pure essential oils and carrier oils of aromatherapy come to us from natural, living and growing plant organisms, and they bear the vital life force that gives true aromatherapy the power to create balance and healing.

Back in 1986, I thought a switch to 'natural' bodycare products would solve my allergy problems, so I rushed out and invested in dozens of 'natural' skincare lotions and oils. To my disappointment, many of these were not much of an improvement over standard, mass-produced cosmetics. I learned to read cosmetic ingredient labels, and discovered that in most cases, so-called 'natural' bases contained the same old synthetic ingredients as standard cosmetics, and caused the same skin reactions. Once aromatherapy became a buzzword, man-made 'aroma-chemical' scents crept into many products as well. While synthetic scents may smell pretty, they have no therapeutic value whatsoever. If you are seriously interested in improving your health and well-being, take the time to learn about truly natural and health-enhancing ingredients and products, and avoid problematic ones, no matter how appealing the packaging or persuasive the advertising surrounding them.

A decade later, I am fortunate to be leading the healthy aromatic life in one of the world's most naturally beautiful areas, the Ojai valley north-west of Los Angeles. As a manufacturer and retailer of true aromatherapy products, I feel blessed to be able to share the education and gifts aromatherapy has given me. Every day, visitors bring us stories of how the practice of true aromatherapy has reduced their stress, improved their health and changed their lives. True aromatherapy is the key that gives natural bodycare its power and veracity. It is my sincere wish that, through these pages, you too will enjoy taking a voyage of discovery into the world of aromatic health and well-being.

Julia Meadows
Ojai, January 1998

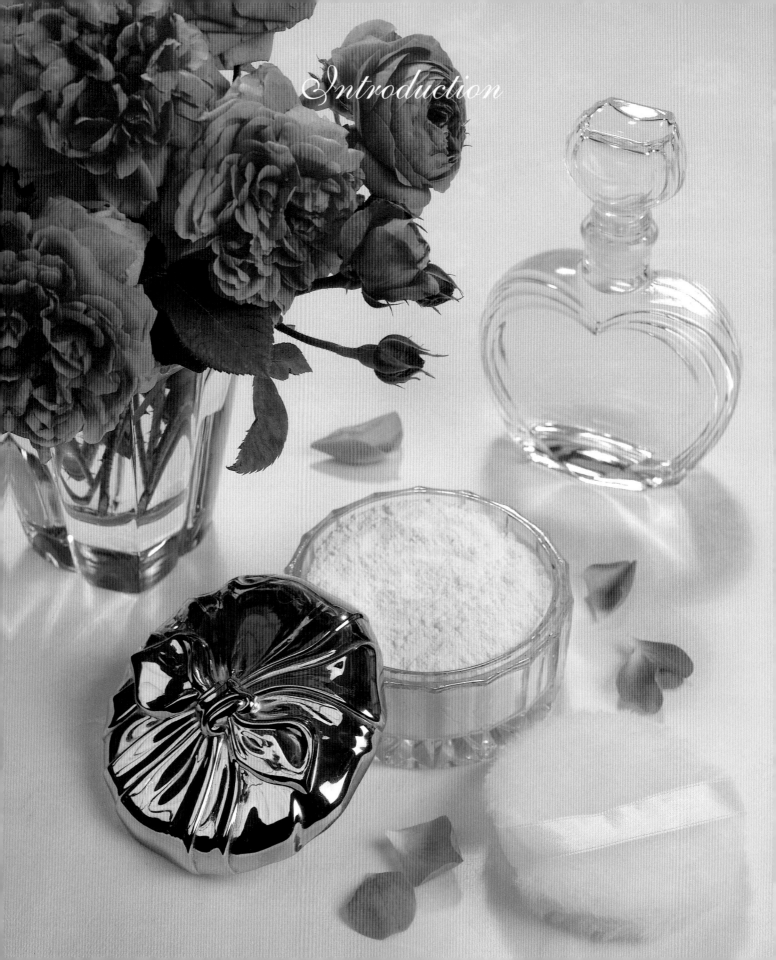

THE DEFINITION OF NATURAL BODYCARE

The subject of natural bodycare has never been more timely, nor more controversial. 'Natural' is the watchword of the 1990's, and the desire for products made from 'natural' ingredients is foremost in consumer consciousness. We believe that natural skincare products, like natural foods and natural healing modalities that have gathered momentum in the past few decades, will improve our beauty, health and well-being in the long term. The clamor for simpler and more effective products having less likelihood of adverse side effects has not been lost on the cosmetic industry. New products come onto the market daily, claiming to offer improved benefits in keeping face and body skin softer, better nourished and more protected from the elements using ingredients derived from Nature.

But how do we define 'natural'? Most people agree with the dictionary definition: "existing in or produced by nature: not artificial." The general consensus is that ingredients that have originated in a living, growing, natural environment are more likely to be well-received by the body than artificial, synthetic compounds which are new and unfamiliar. With over 25,000 cosmetic ingredients currently available to cosmetic formulators, there is no doubt that very few of them are 'natural.' In fact, it is estimated that less than 10% of them can be truly classified as being natural by the dictionary definition. Most are complex mixtures of chemical compounds, whose action is further complicated by their relatively little-known interactions with other chemicals. Much of the debate over 'natural' cosmetics is more than semantic, and goes to the heart of beliefs and experiences. A consumer who is avoiding mineral oil because it causes her skin problems is unlikely to appreciate a cosmetic formulator's argument that the liquid petroleum from which mineral oil is made is natural because fossil fuels are created in the earth by geological pressure. Neither is someone who reacts to synthetic scents with headaches and respiratory problems going to respond favorably to artificially-scented products purporting to provide 'natural,' 'aromatherapy' benefits.

Most of us want products which are natural because we simply believe that they are better for us — milder, healthier, gentler on the skin than mass-produced cosmetics, resulting in fewer adverse reactions. Natural products do fulfill these needs, and

more. But what about issues like stabilization and preservation? Most raw materials that grow in nature or which are derived from natural raw materials face a major problem — they are technically nutrient-rich 'foods' that are very quickly subject to deterioration from micro-organisms and bacteria unless preserved. The vast majority of preservative systems used in commercial cosmetics are of synthetic origin, and these preservatives are included in high concentrations in mass-produced cosmetics so that they can withstand extreme temperature fluctuations and maintain a shelf life of several years. Yet a spoiled or contaminated natural bodycare product is obviously unhealthy and should not be used on the skin. Fortunately, progressive manufacturers are starting to research and work with innovative natural materials, not just those with preservative qualities, but an entire new world of substances, from herbs, vitamins and pure essential oils through to nutritious tropical oils and therapeutic plants originating in developing foreign countries.

In this book, a 'natural' product is defined as one that contains the maximum amount of ingredients derived from the natural plant world which have received only the minimum amount of processing or alteration in order to satisfy health and safety issues, while retaining the ingredients' original, naturally-occurring therapeutic properties. In the case of emulsions, 'natural' means the combination of the least number of basic compounds needed to make a simple and effective preparation, omitting unnecessary chemicals, colors or synthetic fragrance. Within each ingredient category, the simplest and most natural ingredient available is used. Classic examples are the use of cold-pressed oil from nut or seed sources in place of mineral oil, or of organically-grown pure essential oils of botanical origin in place of artificially synthesized 'aroma-chemical' scents. When making your own natural bodycare formulations at home, the issue of whether to preserve them or not is up to you. You may choose to refrigerate non-preserved recipes and use them up quickly, or select between a number of simple preservatives, adding them in low concentrations to your products to ensure a longer shelf life. This book will give you directions and ideas for making a wide array of natural bodycare products, from bath salts, gels and oils to body lotions, creams and perfumes. You will be working with the best ingredients Nature has to offer, creating personalized and healing formulas for yourself, your friends and family — something that cannot be found in any store!

THE MOVEMENT TOWARDS NATURAL HEALTH IN EVERYDAY LIFE

Reasons for developing an interest in the benefits of natural bodycare are many and varied. Many of us, raised in a highly scientific and technological age, are only now discovering the positive aspects of a natural lifestyle and are seeking to incorporate them into our lives to bring balance into our sophisticated, complex world. The rapid advance of scientific progress, while it has brought amazing new developments and conveniences into our lives, has not come without problems — everything from dealing with the side effects of medical and pharmaceutical drugs to re-evaluation of relationships and lifestyles and dealing with greatly increased stress levels. In learning how to care for ourselves better, we are evaluating many positive options available to us, from transformational lifestyle changes through to basic, practical, everyday actions we can take, like making and blending our own personal care products. Our renewed interest in nature stems from the desire to understand, simplify and enjoy our lives more, in a healthy way.

Throughout the industrialized nations generally, people are seeking a simpler life, uncluttered by the material possessions and paraphernalia of previous decades. Social and economic developments have irreversibly changed the way we conduct our personal and business lives. The trend has been away from artificial, towards natural. Pursuits like gardening, herb growing and cooking have soared in popularity in recent years. Architecture, home décor, clothing and entertainment all focus on the expression of natural, simple and personal style. Our new, expanded awareness of holistic mental and physical health is strongly rooted in observing and being in touch with the natural world. Our growing interest in mind/body health and fitness has often led us outdoors, whether to our own gardens or deeper into nature to experience the challenges of hiking and climbing, or simply the joy of being out in the natural world beyond the confines of our working environments.

Since the advent of the ecological 'green' movement in the 1960's, people have begun to feel a greater degree of control over their working and personal lives, from the foods they eat to the products they use daily. The 'back to basics' movement of those days is resurfacing in a different form as people begin to educate themselves more and more on matters of consumer interest and make their preferences known. The current move-

ment towards alternative medicine is a powerful example of this. Natural therapies are being sought out by increasing numbers of people who are disenchanted with traditional allopathic medical practice, and a wide variety of modalities are becoming mainstream. Consumer interest in nutritional supplements, anti-aging compounds and botanicals has reached an all-time high. Rather than trusting blindly in conventional medicine, many people are now taking active responsibility for their own health and longevity.

Diet, exercise, meditation and other elements of the natural lifestyle fit into this self-care equation. For the first time in history, people are willing to pay a premium for access to health-giving items such as exercise equipment, spa memberships and organically-grown produce. Farmers' markets are more popular than ever; natural foods stores have experienced tremendous growth; even conventional supermarkets have greatly expanded their repertoire to cater to an aware and health-conscious public. With increasing frequency, people are taking vacations at new 'destination' spas and resorts that offer extensive menus of mind/body healing services and treatments. The famous Latin phrase 'mens sana in corpore sano' — a healthy mind in a healthy body — is becoming a pre-millennium credo. Now that the average life-span has increased dramatically, we want to achieve optimum health and well-being in order to enjoy our extra time on the planet.

CHANGING THE WAY WE WORK AND LIVE

Along with our extended lifespans, we want to be able to look forward to lifestyles that are pleasurable, rewarding and productive. With the concept of the nuclear family irreversibly changed, most of our extended family relationships, friendships and partnerships are now radically different. Our interactions with work colleagues and business associates have been similarly altered by corporate readjustment and downsizing, by the advent of computer technology and the development of the global economy. These changes have led many to seek out a deeper community and social involvement as well as fostering personal individuality and uniqueness. Having re-evaluated their lives, many people want to make the time to take a 'hands-on' approach to subjects that interest them. As a result, personal expression can be seen in the formation of home-based businesses and the development of hobbies into small-scale commercial ventures. Increasingly, people are taking personal pleasure in learning and mastering a new skill, particularly one with its roots in history or tradition. The herbal, bodywork and natural arts and crafts traditions of many countries around the world are in the spotlight. Whether for fun or profit, traditional methods and materials are being re-interpreted and presented to a receptive audience. Added to this is the personal pleasure of creating custom products for oneself as well as heart-felt and health-giving natural gifts for family and friends. As these newly-discovered materials and techniques become more widely disseminated, more and more people are able to experience for themselves how healthy, cost-effective and enjoyable they are, choosing to include their favorites into their everyday lives.

THE TREND TOWARDS SIMPLE, HONEST AND COST-EFFECTIVE COSMETICS

As with natural therapies, people are now much more aware of their options in selecting and purchasing products that will positively affect their general well-being. Today's consumers expect a fair return on the money, time and energy they invest in material goods, whether they are household items or personal luxuries. Cosmetic products in particular have come under close scrutiny. While advertising remains a powerful force, people now want to know what ingredients are in a product, why they are there, and what they are expected to accomplish. Nowadays, products that do not perform to expectations are unlikely to have a long lifespan in a market saturated with personal care products. Consumers have the luxury of picking and choosing between more products than ever before, and informed purchasing is growing exponentially.

Money is another factor governing the interest in natural skincare products. The cost of many commercial skincare offerings, particularly moisturizers and creams promising near-miracu-lous results, is frequently perceived to be too high in compari-son to the actual results obtained. Consumers are aware that a great percentage of the cost of a specialty cosmetic such as an 'anti-aging' cream lies not in the ingredients, but in the excessive packaging, glamorized advertising and associated sales and distribution costs. Consumers are starting to ask for more proof of the claims made for a specific product. People can now often find more effective, natural skincare products at other specialty retail outlets and through mail order at a lower cost, and with more consumer support. In addition, the increased availability of a wide range of economical natural ingredients has enabled people to view making their own personal care products as a cost-effective and attractive option.

Freshness and authenticity of product ingredients is also a concern. People want to select from an exciting range of new ingredients now available to them, and they want products that are sufficiently customized to enable the new ingredients to provide their special qualities directly. Commercial cosmetic companies have to prepare their products for a standardized market, and so cannot address the needs of customization very easily. Over the past decade, demand for fresh and organic goods has driven the natural food industry to adopt 'freshness dating' — an 'expiry date' by which time the product should be con-sumed for optimum health results. Cosmetic manufacturers, suppliers and retailers are not able to provide this service for skincare products, as it would amount to a logistical nightmare for existing distribution and operation systems. Some progressive bodycare companies have begun to identify the time-sensitive nature of their natural products with 'best before' dates, but this practice is relatively new and not yet widespread. In order to make a completely fresh, natural product that is customized to meet specific skincare needs, it is necessary to make it right at home.

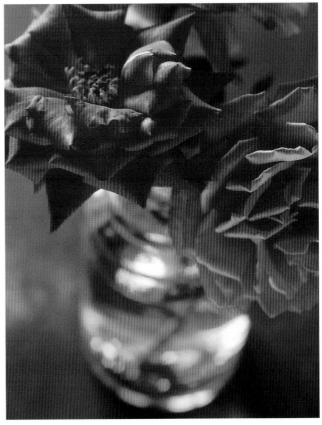

Many people are interested in making their own bodycare formulations because they have skin sensitivities, have experienced problems with mass-produced products in the past and are unable to find other products on the market which don't include the particular ingredients they are sensitive to. Many have found that their usual skincare products are not working as well as previously, that their skin has stopped responding, or worse, that it is starting to react negatively to a product that worked before. In some cases, individuals have developed reactions to some products, resulting in a variety of responses from a vague headachy feeling through to a full-blown allergy. If you are under great stress and your immune system is temporarily affected, exposure to the chemicals and synthetic fragrances present in many mass-produced products will certainly not help your condition and should be minimized or avoided.

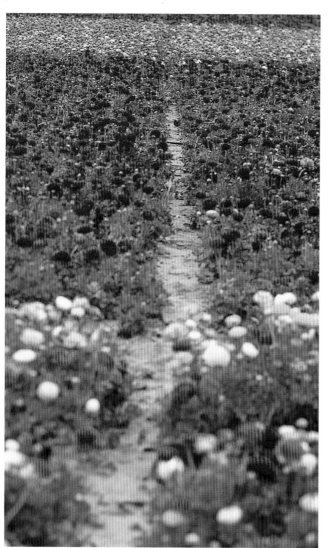

One of the most problematic cosmetic categories for the sensitive or allergy-prone are synthetic fragrance compounds ('aroma-chemicals.') Virtually every mass-produced household and cosmetic product on the market contains synthetic fragrance, even 'unscented' products that contain 'masking' fragrances to cover the odor of the product ingredients! Possibly the biggest misinformation provided to consumers in recent years is the fallacy that synthetically-fragranced products will somehow have physiological and psychological 'aromatherapy' effects. While one might have a brief, pleasant associative connection with a synthetic scent, the fact remains that aroma-chemical compounds derived from petrochemical sources are artificial substances that are alien to the body. The proliferation of scents found nowhere in nature, while acceptable in perfumery and cosmetics, offers no therapeutic or health-promoting value to those seeking truly natural solutions to their skincare needs. In order to have true aromatherapeutic value, only premium-quality pure essential oils of botanical origin should be used in natural bodycare products for their fragrant and healing properties.

THE ADVENT OF TRUE AROMATHERAPY FOR HEALTH AND BEAUTY

Aromatherapy has become a global buzzword in recent years, yet public awareness of its benefits is still limited, largely as a result of misleading advertising and inaccurate product labeling by cosmetic companies wanting to capitalize on the healing abilities of this ancient art. Simply stated, true aromatherapy is the use of the pure essential oils of plants, herbs and flowers in health and beauty products and treatments to produce a healing, regulating or balancing effect. The true aromatherapy formulas in this book focus on combining pure essential oils from botanical sources with simple natural ingredients, herbs and vitamins to create natural products that will foster your health and beauty while providing nourishment for body, mind and soul. Once you become familiar with true aromatherapy, there will be no turning back! Your senses will be awakened and heightened, and you'll become increasingly aware of the many ways in which Nature provides us with all we need for maintaining and enhancing wellness. True aromatherapy provides its benefits in the most pleasurable and sensual ways — through inhalation, massage and application of rich and wonderful natural aromas that nurture and heal. In order to fully understand the benefits of essential oils, it's useful to know about their historical uses, origins and effects on the body/mind.

Aromatherapy has been known and practiced for centuries. The early civilizations — Egyptian, Greek, Roman, Chinese, Indian — all made use of aromatic plant materials in religious ritual, for healing, and to promote physical and mental well-being. Throughout the centuries, essential oils have had healing applications in the herbal tradition, but the word 'aromatherapy' was not coined until the 1930's, when several European doctors and biochemists integrated their essential oil research into their work. Aromatherapy, when properly practiced, has shown successful results in the treatment of muscular, circulatory, respiratory, digestive and reproductive problems, as well as skin disorders and stress-related conditions. Although rooted in ancient history, pure essential oils offer revolutionary new benefits to the practice and effectiveness of natural bodycare.

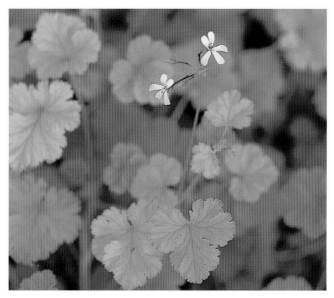

Pure essential oils are obtained from the leaves, branches, flowers, roots and barks of plants, as well as spices and the rinds of citrus fruits. As they occur naturally in plants, their quality is largely determined by a range of factors including place of origin, plant type, geographic locale, cultivation methods, climatic changes and distillation techniques. The majority of essential oils are obtained from plants by steam distillation, producing a volatile 'oil' (e.g., lavender, geranium.) Citrus oils are obtained by 'expression' — cold-pressing the fruit peel mechanically or by hand (e.g., lemon, grapefruit.) Some aromatic materials, such as concretes and absolutes (e.g., rose, jasmine) are made from highly fragrant flowers whose petals are too delicate for steam distillation. Absolutes are created from flower materials through the use of solvents that are later washed with alcohol to remove them, leaving the fragrant 'absolute.' Oleoresins, resinoids and

balsams are a further classification of natural aromatic materials obtained from gums, resins and woods (e.g., benzoin, myrrh.) These processes all result in fragrant plant 'essences' — natural liquids with the characteristic aroma and properties of the plant from which they were obtained.

Essential oils affect the body and mind in various ways. Inhalation of the essential oils, either directly or with the use of a diffuser, is the most immediate. Ambient or environmental aromatherapy is achieved through the use of essential oils with dispersing equipment such as nebulizers and electric or ceramic diffusers. Drops can also be inhaled directly from a tissue or placed on sachets or natural potpourris to freshen the air and provide aromatherapy benefits. The practice of using essential oils to influence mood through inhalation is called 'psycho-aromatherapy.' Blending essential oils into a carrier oil base and applying them to the body, face and scalp with massage techniques is at the heart of the practice of true aromatherapy. In addition to carrier oil bases, essential oils can easily be mixed with lotions, gels, salts, powders and other natural bases for use in body and skincare products. It is believed that, much like transdermal medications and liposomes, the active ingredients in essential oils have the ability to penetrate the skin. When the appropriate essential oils are chosen, they have the ability to stimulate or relax, normalize skin metabolism, correct imbalances and generally regulate and improve the body's functions. For natural skin and bodycare, many essential oils are available which have remarkable anti-bacterial, anti-inflammatory, regulating and cytophylactic (cell-regenerating) properties.

The formulas in this book have been especially created to give you an introduction to the fragrant and healing world of true aromatherapy. Some of the recipes contain herbs in combination with essential oils, and nutrient-rich natural oils and anti-oxidant vitamins are included in others. The recipes use the simplest, most healthful ingredients possible to help you realize the beauty and health potential of these time-tested, ageless gifts of Nature. You will be amazed at the versatility, gentleness and effectiveness of essential oils in combination with other natural bodycare ingredients. You'll gain the ability to customize formulas for yourself, your friends and family, adapting them to meet specific needs as your health and beauty needs change. You will be acting as your own cosmetic formulator, manufacturer and quality control expert, and you'll experience the excitement of seeing the positive results of your new skills. Welcome to the world of natural bodycare!

Chapter One
Ingredients

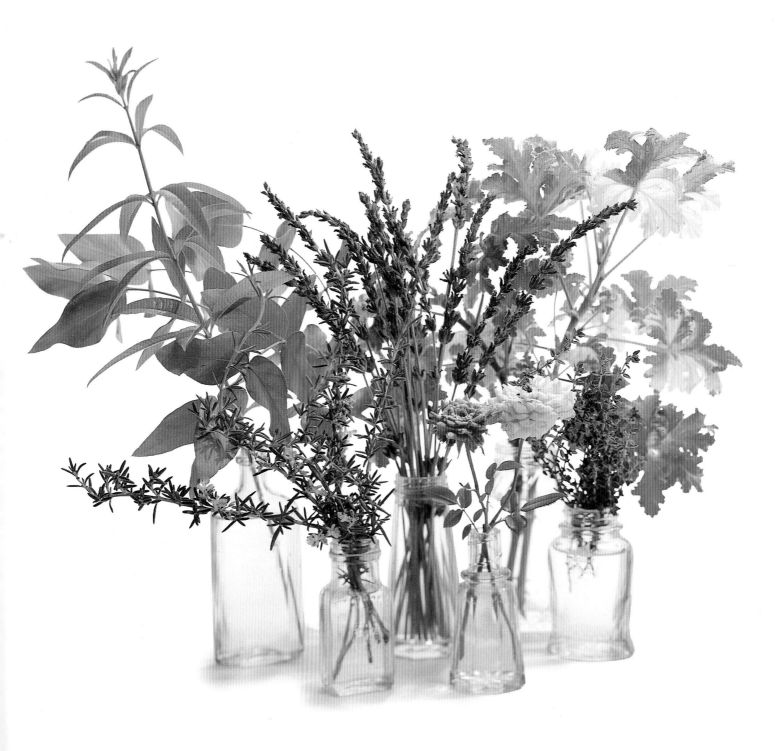

Introduction to Natural Ingredients

This chapter is designed to give you an overview of the ingredients you'll be using to create your own natural bodycare products at home. For easy reference, this section is divided into nine categories of ingredients with photographs accompanying each one. Because homemade recipes and remedies have traditionally used simple household materials as cosmetic ingredients, you may be surprised how many of these ingredients you already have at home. Almost everyone will recognize the natural materials described in the 'Liquid Ingredients,' 'Dry Materials,' 'Nut, Grain and Fruit Ingredients' and 'Ingredients from the Kitchen' categories. In the past few years, due largely to the cosmetic industry's interest in developing 'natural' formulas, new categories of ingredients have entered the limelight. Some of these are old-fashioned, tried and true substances, like 'Herbal Ingredients' and 'Plant Butters and Waxes,' while others come from the relatively new art and science of true aromatherapy,including 'Carrier Oils' and 'Pure Essential Oils, Absolutes and Oleoresins.' The final category, 'Cosmetic Ingredients,' includes vitamins, preservatives and ingredients used in modern natural skincare products.

This book focuses on the most important herbs, essential oils and natural ingredients specifically used in skincare, enabling you to become familiar with each one in order to be able to judge quality when you are shopping for ingredients. The ingredients outlined here are available from a wide range of suppliers; from supermarkets, drugstores and natural foods stores, to specialty retailers, scientific supply houses and specialized mail order suppliers. If you have any difficulty obtaining any ingredient listed here, contact the resource address given on page 125.

A word about preservation: if your natural products contain fresh ingredients such as fruit, milk or eggs, you will probably want to use them right away. Other products, particularly lotions and creams, will need to be preserved if

you want to keep them for some time. Preservation is defined as the addition of anti-bacterial, anti-fungal, anti-viral and anti-microbial substances to a compound that would otherwise quickly spoil and decay. Contamination of food-grade, nutrient rich compounds by pathogenic micro-organisms is inevitable if they are not preserved, so the FDA and the cosmetic industry consider preservation of cosmetic products a necessity in protecting public health. You can choose to preserve your products with lesser amounts of more natural preservatives in order to obtain a reasonable shelf life. If you would like to preserve your home products, be sure to include effective substances such as grapefruit seed extract, a non-toxic natural preservative compound. To give an extended shelf life to creams and lotions, another alternative is Germaben II, a broad-spectrum preservative containing parabens and diazolidinyl urea, which has been found to be mild and non-irritating while exhibiting excellent preservative qualities.

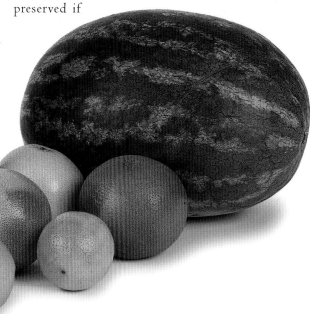

Liquid Ingredients

Water: The major component of all living things, water is also usually the main ingredient in many bodycare formulas. Distilled water and spring water are both suitable for use in oil/water emulsions.

Herbal teas and infusions: To add the specific therapeutic qualities of botanicals to your recipes, use herb teas and infusions in place of water.

Mineral water: Sparkling mineral water adds a clean, revitalizing element to custom-made facial recipes, toners and specialty treatments. Mineral waters refresh, detoxify and relax the skin.

Milk: Milk is rich in proteins, calcium and vitamins, and is excellent for bathing and for facial skincare. Whole milk is most nutritious for the skin as it contains a high percentage of butterfat.

Orange flower water: This naturally fragrant water is distilled from the blossoms of the bitter orange tree. Excellent for skincare, orange flower water is cleansing and slightly astringent.

Rose water: Originating in Persia centuries ago, rose water is distilled from fresh rose petals. The clear, mild, delicately perfumed water is an excellent cleanser, humectant and moisturizer.

Aloe vera gel: The tropical aloe vera plant (Aloe barbadensis) has fleshy leaves which contain a cool, transparent gel full of nutrients which promote healing and skin cell renewal. A soothing natural anti-inflammatory and moisturizer.

Witch hazel: Branches of the shrub (Hamamelis virginiana) when distilled yield a clear liquid extract which is excellent for cleansing and toning the skin.

Alcohol: Alcohol is clarifying and astringent and is used for its solvent and preservative effects in natural skincare formulations. Use 90-proof unflavored vodka in your recipes. Alcohol is used in herbal tinctures and to disperse essential oils.

Apple cider vinegar: Fermented vinegars have been used in bodycare for over 5,000 years. Apple cider vinegar helps restore skin's natural pH balanced acid mantle.

Vegetable glycerin: A clear, odorless, thick and slightly sticky liquid that holds moisture to the skin and is readily absorbed, imparting a smooth, silky feel.

Lemon juice: Fresh-squeezed lemon juice with pulp and seeds removed is used in skincare recipes to cleanse, tone, destroy bacteria, and regulate the pH factor of the skin.

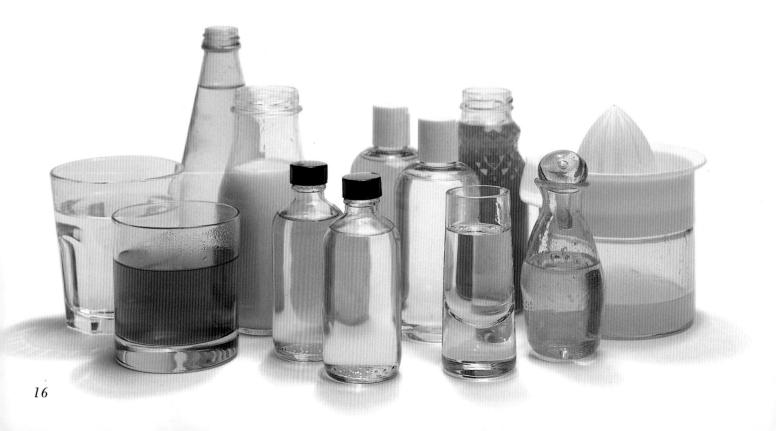

Ingredients from the Kitchen

Extracts and flavorings: Natural flavorings can be used when you want a light, sweet aromatic fragrance in an alcohol base to add to recipes. Natural extracts include vanilla, almond and certain fruits.

Almonds: The nuts of the almond tree (Prunus dulcis) have been used cosmetically for centuries. Sweet almond oil is cold-pressed from the nuts, while the nutritious ground meal is excellent for facial scrubs.

Brown sugar: Raw, turbinado or demerara sugars all make a simple and effective organic exfoliating material. Mix sugar with liquid gel bases to make an all-natural body scrub.

Yogurt: Unflavored cultured yogurt contains beneficial lactobacilli which destroy bacteria on the skin. Yogurt makes an excellent base for mixing herb powders and essential oils. Try it in face and body masks.

Cream: Ideal for dry, dehydrated or flaking skins, rich cream is exceptionally high in protein, calcium and fats. Use it in cleansers and bath recipes and see how smooth and soft your skin feels.

Oats: (Avena sativa) Oats have been used cosmetically for centuries. Oatmeal, oat bran and oat flour each have therapeutic qualities when added to natural recipes.

Lemon and citrus fruits: All parts of citrus fruits — the rind, peel and juices — are used either fresh or dried in natural recipes. Their anti-bacterial acid content and fresh fragrance are particularly useful in natural skincare.

Homemade mayonnaise: A natural mayonnaise made with egg, oil and lemon is one of the most nutritious skin conditioners you can create. Pure essential oils add fragrance and therapeutic value.

Honey: Made from the nectar of flowering plants by bees, honey has been a staple in beauty products for centuries. Honey is a powerhouse of vitamins, minerals, amino acids and enzymes, making it a unique and versatile skincare ingredient. Bacteria cannot live in honey, demonstrating its natural preservative properties.

Powdered milk: Dehydrated milk makes an excellent absorbent carrier material for herbal powders and essential oils in bath preparations.

Eggs: Fresh eggs have been used throughout history to soften and nourish skin. Egg whites (albumen) have a tightening effect on the skin, while egg yolks are rich in protein and vitamins and are used in facial and hair conditioning treatments.

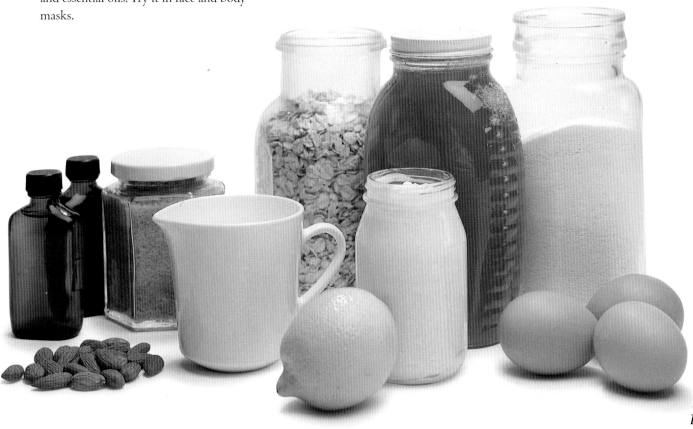

Dry Ingredients

Sea salts: The basis for bath salts as well as detoxifying body scrubs and spa treatments, sea salts are available in fine and coarse grades. Look for naturally-dried salts (preferably solar-dried) which have not been chemically-treated.

Epsom salts: (Magnesium sulfate) Epsom salts have been used for years in the bath to alleviate muscular aches and pains and arthritic conditions. They are also very effective when added to a warm footbath. They make an excellent addition to bath salt recipes.

Borax: (Sodium tetraborate) A mild alkaline salt mined in the western U.S. Borax has water-softening abilities and is used as a texturizer and preservative in creams, lotions and salves.

Flowers of sulfur: This bright yellow powder has been used for decades to make an astringent paste to dry up blemishes and acne.

Clays: Various types of cosmetic clays exist which have slightly different therapeutic effects in skincare depending on their unique mineral content. Rich in trace elements, clays have been used since ancient times to cleanse and detoxify the body. Use them in mud packs for face, body and haircare.

Sea clay: A particularly mineral-rich dark green clay which is obtained from the ocean floor. It has a high seaweed and algae content which makes it ideal for purifying and toning body treatments.

Herbal powders: Ground powders that are easily incorporated into product bases are a convenient way to experience the active healing properties of herbs.

Xanthan gum: This powdery white substance is a polysaccharide (natural sugar) produced by carbohydrate fermentation. It is used in natural bodycare recipes as a thickener, stabilizer and emulsifier.

Arrowroot powder: A starch derived from plant roots, arrowroot is used in cosmetics as a carrier medium and as a natural ingredient in body dusting powders.

Cornstarch: A fine white powder, that, like rice starch and arrowroot powder, is a neutral carrier ingredient for use in natural dusting powders.

Flours: Fine-ground flours to use in natural bodycare recipes include oat, rice and potato flours. All act as gentle bulking agents and can be included in face and body powders and used to thicken fruit and vegetable juices for clarifying facial treatments.

Nut, Grain and Fruit Peel Ingredients

Almond meal: Fine-ground almonds provide a highly nutritious 'meal' that has been used for centuries as cleansing grains in scrubs for face and body skin. Almond meal is particularly rich in vitamins, minerals and beneficial oils.

Cornmeal: Yellow cornmeal makes an excellent scrub ingredient for oilier skins. It has a dense consistency and great absorbent qualities, and is popular in spa treatments as a key ingredient in purifying full-body exfoliation treatments.

Orange peel: Citrus peels of all kinds — orange, lemon, mandarin, grapefruit and lime — make excellent fresh or dried cleansing grains. If used fresh, add them to carrier bases just prior to treatment; if used dried, pulverize them thoroughly in a nut grinder to a fine consistency.

Oatmeal: A classic ingredient for skin and bodycare, oats can be ground to a variety of consistencies for use in scrubs, masks, or as soothing bath grains. Oats contain amino acids and trace elements that are highly soothing to inflamed, irritated and itchy skin.

Ground coffee: Fine-ground coffee beans, when added to scrubs, have a detoxifying and invigorating effect on the skin and provide gentle but thorough exfoliation.

Psyllium husks: A lightweight yet slightly abrasive material that is a good additive to scrubs for oily or blemish-prone skin. Psyllium husks purify the skin and remove dead skin cells and excess oil.

Black walnut hulls: The fine, hard grains of pulverized black walnuts make a gritty and abrasive material that can be added to liquid soap or lotion bases to make an effective hand or foot scrub cleanser.

Wheat bran: A nutritious and skin-softening ingredient in face and body scrubs. Add it to carrier bases just before treatment for best results.

Ground orris root: Typically used as a fixative in natural pot-pourris, ground orris root is used in dusting powders, sachets and occasionally as a cleansing scrub material.

Amaranth: A small, smooth grain best known as a breakfast cereal, amaranth, when added to carrier bases, makes an excellent non-abrasive material for an all-over body polish treatment.

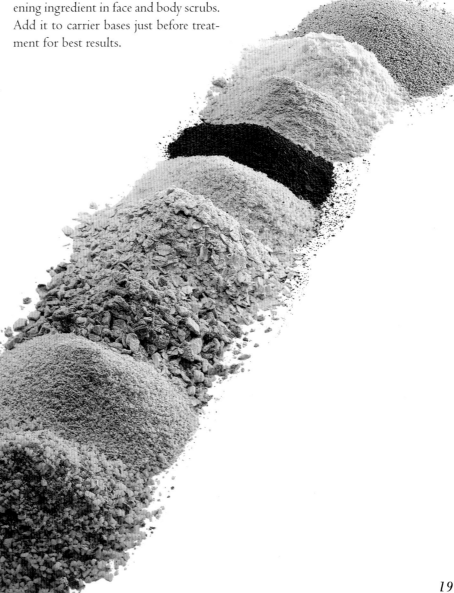

Plant Butters and Waxes

Shea butter: (Butyrospermum parkii) This cream-colored plant butter is obtained from the nuts of the bassia parkii tree that grows along the west coast of Africa. It is an excellent cosmetic ingredient as it contains Vitamins A and E, known for their anti-oxidant and skin-nourishing effects, and the healing substance allantoin. Cinnamic esters in shea butter also provide natural protection from UV rays. Shea butter's creamy and deep-moisturizing texture makes it an invaluable addition to high-quality face and hand creams. It is also known as 'karite' butter.

Cocoa butter: (Theobroma cacao) Although native to South America, the cocoa tree grows in all tropical countries. Cocoa butter is obtained from the roasted seeds from which cocoa and chocolate are made. Cocoa 'beans' are composed of 40 – 50% fats that after processing yield a waxy, pale yellow material with a slightly sweet, chocolate-like aroma. Cocoa butter has been used in the confectionery, pharmaceutical and cosmetic industries for years, and it is compatible with a wide range of raw materials, including plant oils and essential oils. It is very effective as an emollient, and is used in creams and salves to soften and soothe the skin.

Beeswax: The classic wax for use in face creams, salves and solid perfumes. Bees process honey from nectar and then convert it into wax (one pound of wax is made from each ten pounds of honey). Beeswax is available in natural (yellow) and bleached (white) forms in blocks, or granulated into beads for easier use. Melt beeswax in a 'bain marie' to make it liquid for natural bodycare recipes. It acts as an emulsifying agent and makes an excellent clean and bacteria-resistant base for your cosmetic recipes.

Carnauba wax: Both carnauba wax and candelilla waxes, from tropical plant sources, are used to make cosmetic creams, lip salves and solid perfumes. Available in flake form, add a pinch of wax to add gloss and shine to your cosmetic products.

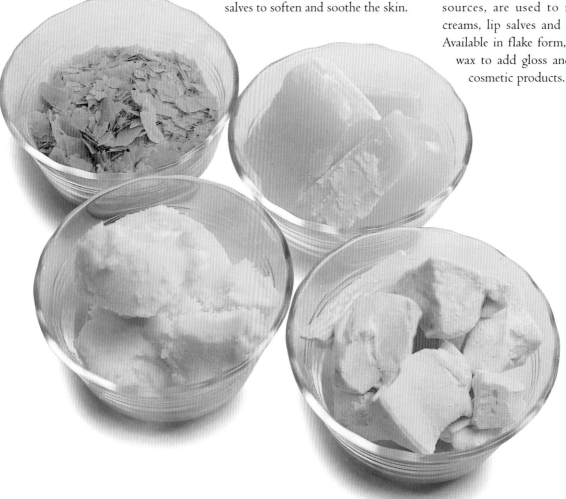

Herbal Ingredients

Rose petals: (Rosa damascena/Rosa centifolia) Roses have a strong tradition in skincare. The petals and buds are used both fresh and dried for their softening and toning effects on dry and sensitive skin. Fragrant pink and red rose petals are also used to make rosewater.

Lavender: (Lavendula angustifolia/ Lavendula vera) Lavender has been used for centuries to freshen rooms and fragrance the air. The aroma of its purplish-blue flowers seems to intensify when dried. Lavender flowers have traditionally been used in sachets, sleep pillows and natural pot-pourris.

Chamomile: (Chamaemelum nobile/ Chamomilla recutita) Infusion of chamomile has been used for generations to soothe nerves, settle stomachs and induce restful sleep. The dried flowers contain potent anti-inflammatory substances and are used externally to care for dry or mature facial skin, especially the area around the eyes.

Lemon verbena: (Aloysia triphylla/ Lippia citriodora) The tangy, lemon-scented leaves of this shrub have always been popular for pot-pourris and sachets. When infused, lemon verbena leaves make a light, refreshing tea that can also be used in place of water in recipes for normal to oily skin types.

Calendula/marigold: (Calendula officinalis) Renowned for its healing abilities, calendula is a soothing antiseptic and an excellent skin healer. Its bright orange petals have been used for centuries to make an infused oil for skincare.

Elder flower: (Sambucus nigra) The elder tree was once called "the medicine chest of the common people." The sweet-smelling flowers are used to make elder flower water for washing the complexion as well as salves and ointments for bruises and sprains.

Peppermint: (Mentha piperita) The best known member of the mint family, peppermint, has a clean, invigorating aroma when dried. Peppermint infusion makes a cooling and refreshing wash for normal to oily skin types. It makes a great aromatic tonic to relieve a headache, and is a popular ingredient in hand and foot lotions.

Lemongrass: (Cymbopogon citratus) This tropical grass grows six feet tall and has a wonderful lemon fragrance. Lemongrass can be dried and made into an infusion for inclusion in recipes for oily skin. It is reputed to improve tired and sagging skin.

Sage: (Salvia officinalis) Sage is a potent herb whose leaves can be infused to produce a strong-scented tea that is used as a complexion wash for oily skin, a hair tonic or shampoo, and a cleansing, purifying and deodorizing body wash.

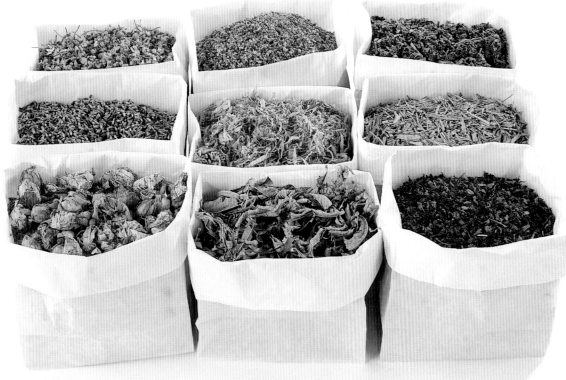

Pure Essential Oils, Absolutes and Oleo-Resins

Lavender: (Lavandula angustifolia/ Lavandula vera) Lavender is considered to be the most versatile essential oil in the aromatherapy repertoire. It has a distinctive fresh, clean aroma and is known for its soothing and healing properties in skincare.

Chamomile: (Chamaemelum nobile) A beautiful blue-tinged oil, Roman chamomile contains potent anti-inflammatory substances and is recommended for use in cases of dry, irritated or inflamed skin and for the treatment of eczema and skin rashes.

Geranium: (Pelargonium graveolens) Distilled from the leaves of the scented geranium, this yellow oil with a greenish tinge has a clean, rosy-floral aroma and is known for its ability to balance and regulate skin functions,

Tea Tree: (Melaleuca alternifolia) A clear oil derived from the leaves of bushes grown mostly in Australia, tea tree oil contains valuable anti-bacterial compounds which cleanse and detoxify oily or blemished skin.

Cedarwood Atlas: (Cedrus atlantica) This light golden oil has a warm, woodsy aroma and blends well with citrus oils. Cedarwood is a balancing and normalizing oil that is a good addition to formulas for normal to oily skin types.

Jasmine: (Jasminum officinale) Jasmine absolute is extracted from the flowers and is a thick, deep reddish-brown liquid with a wonderful, rich aroma. Very few drops are needed to impart its aroma and therapeutic values into skincare recipes for all skin types.

Rosemary: (Rosmarinus officinalis) A clear, bright oil, rosemary has a strong camphoraceous aroma typical of the herb. It is classically paired with lavender in bodycare recipes and has an energizing, tonic effect on the skin.

Grapefruit: (Citrus paradisi) Grapefruit oil is pale yellow with a slight pinkish tinge and a sweet, crisp aroma exactly like fresh grapefruit. The oil of choice for cellulite reduction, grapefruit is also good for treating oily, congested skin.

Rose: (Rosa damascena/Rosa centifolia) Rose absolute is the most effective oil for facial skincare, particularly for dry or mature skin types. The absolute has a warm amber color and the distinctive, heady aroma of full-blown roses.

Lemon: (Citrus limon) Lemon oil has a clean, distinctive aroma just like the newly-peeled fruit. A revitalizing and energizing oil for skincare, particularly for oily skin.

Vanilla: (Vanilla planifolia) Technically an oleoresin, real vanilla is extracted from the ripened bean pod and is a thick, rich brown liquid. Its warm and comforting aroma is welcome in all bodycare formulas, and it blends well with most essential oils.

Sweet orange: (Citrus sinensis) Orange oil has a sparkling greenish-orange color and warm and cheerful aroma characteristic of the ripe fruit. A versatile oil which gives its sweet fragrance and normalizing therapeutic values to bodycare recipes for all skin types.

Mandarin: (Citrus reticulata) A warm, deliciously fruity, orange-colored oil with a characteristic aroma, mandarin oil is a welcome addition to bodycare recipes.

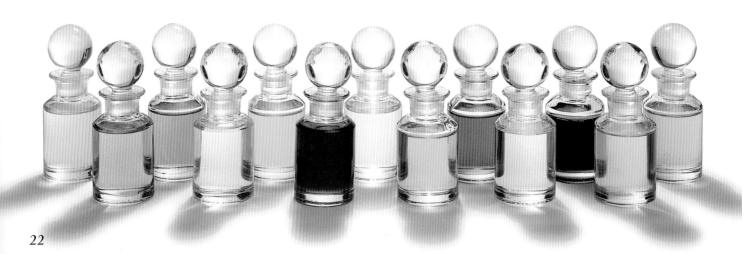

Pure Essential Oils for Natural Bodycare

ESSENTIAL OIL	BOTANICAL NAME	PLANT PART	NOTE
BASIL	*Ocimum basilicum*	Flowering tops	M
BENZOIN**	*Styrax benzoin*	Resin	B
BERGAMOT	*Citrus bergamia*	Rind of fruit	T
CEDARWOOD ATLAS	*Cedrus atlantica*	Wood	B
CHAMOMILE, GERMAN	*Chamomilla recutita*	Flowers	M
CHAMOMILE, ROMAN	*Chamaemelum nobile*	Flowers	M
CLARY SAGE	*Salvia sclarea*	Flowering tops	M
CYPRESS	*Cupressus sempervirens*	Leaf	M
EUCALYPTUS	*Eucalyptus globulus*	Leaf	T
FRANKINCENSE	*Boswellia carterii*	Resinous gum	B
GERANIUM	*Pelargonium graveolens*	Flowering tops	M
GRAPEFRUIT	*Citrus paradisi*	Rind of fruit	T
JASMINE*	*Jasminum officinale*	Flowers	B
JUNIPER BERRY	*Juniperus communis*	Berry	M
LAVENDER	*Lavendula angustifolia*	Flowering tops	M
LEMON	*Citrus limonum*	Rind of fruit	T
MANDARIN	*Citrus reticulata*	Rind of fruit	T
MELISSA	*Melissa officinalis*	Flowering tops	M
MYRHH	*Commiphora myrhha*	Resinous gum	B
NEROLI	*Citrus aurantium bigarade*	Flowers	M
ORANGE, SWEET	*Citrus aurantium var. dulcis*	Rind of fruit	T
PALMAROSA	*Cymbopogon martinii*	Grass	M
PATCHOULI	*Pogostemon cablin*	Leaf	B
PEPPERMINT	*Mentha piperita*	Leaf	T
PETITGRAIN	*Citrus aurantium var. amara*	Leaf/Branch	T
PINE, SCOTCH	*Pinus sylvestris*	Leaf	M
ROSE*	*Rosa damascena*	Flowers	B
ROSEMARY	*Rosmarinus officinalis*	Flowering tops	T
ROSEWOOD	*Ocotea caudata*	Wood	B
SAGE, SPANISH	*Salvia lavendulaefolia*	Flowering tops	M
SANDALWOOD	*Santalum album*	Wood	B
TEA TREE	*Melaleuca alternifolia*	Leaf	M
THYME, WHITE	*Thymus vulgaris*	Flowering tops	M
VALERIAN	*Valeriana officinalis*	Root	B
VANILLA**	*Vanilla planifolia*	Seed pod	B
VERBENA	*Aloysia triphylla*	Leaf	T
YLANG YLANG	*Cananga odorata genuina*	Flower	M

* Absolute ** Oleoresin

T = Top Note M = Middle Note B = Base Note

Carrier Oils

Sweet almond: (Prunus dulcis) The most popular oil for aromatherapy massage and general skincare, sweet almond oil is a mild, straw-colored oil that is nutrient-rich and is suitable for all skin types.

Grapeseed: (Vitis vinifera) A green-tinted oil much used in massage and skincare, grapeseed oil is produced from the seeds of wine-producing grapes. A fine-textured oil that is nourishing for all skin types.

Hazelnut: (Corylus avellana) Hazelnuts contain over 60% of an oil that, like sweet almond oil, is excellent for face, scalp and bodycare use. A golden-colored oil with a light, sweet aroma and smooth texture.

Pecan: (Carya illinoinensis) Pecan is a member of the walnut family that produces a highly nutritious pale golden oil for skincare. Pecan oil is recommended for all skin types.

Avocado: (Persea americana) A rich greenish oil with a high content of protein, Vitamins A and E and the 'youth mineral', potassium. Avocado oil is especially valued when a rich, nourishing oil is needed in skincare, particularly to treat dry, dehydrated or damaged skin. Avocado oil is excellent in hair and scalp formulas.

Jojoba: (Simmondsia chinensis) Technically a 'liquid wax,' jojoba has a comparatively large molecular structure and lasts much longer than other carrier oils without becoming rancid. Jojoba is a popular oil that is frequently used for hair and scalp care. For bodycare, it is best blended with lighter oils.

Wheatgerm: (Triticum vulgare) A deep orange oil with a characteristic strong smell, wheatgerm is a rich source of Vitamin E and essential fatty acids. Wheatgerm oil by itself is thick and sticky, but when blended with other oils it imparts a rich satiny feel and, being antioxidant, has an extended shelf life. Wheatgerm oil is an excellent addition to facial oil blends.

Evening primrose: (Oenethera biennis) Evening primrose oil has been the subject of extensive research, as it is one of the few plant sources of GLA (gamma-linoleic acid) that has many therapeutic applications both internally and in natural skincare. A pale yellow oil, it blends well with other carrier oils to make a superior oil for bodycare.

Carrot root: (Daucus carota) Not to be confused with carrot seed essential oil, carrot root oil is the rich golden oil obtained from the carrots themselves. High in Vitamin A and beta-carotene, carrot oil is a healing addition to facial oils for dry or mature skin.

Calendula: (Calendula officinalis) Infused oil of calendula is made by steeping the bright yellow or orange flower petals in oil. Calendula has a historical reputation for healing wounds and soothing skin eruptions, eczema and rough, chapped and damaged skin.

St. John's Wort: (Hypericum perforatum) An oil with a fascinating and symbolic history, infused oil of St. John's Wort is a ruby red color and has been used since the Middle Ages to reduce muscular pain and relieve skin conditions of nervous origin.

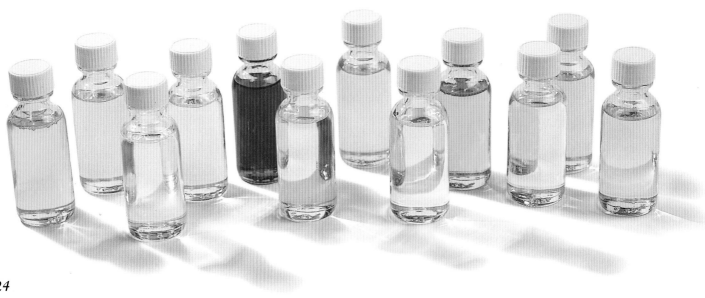

Cosmetic Ingredients

Distilled water: The primary ingredient in many formulations, distilled water is free of the mineral salts and metals that are present in ordinary tap water.

Polyglucose/sucrose cocoate: Manufactured from glucose (sugar) and fatty acids, polyglucose and sucrose cocoate are mild, biodegradable surfactants ('surface active agents') suitable for making gels.

Coco betaine: Made from coconut oil, coco betaine is a mild biodegradable surfactant with cleansing, foaming and emulsifying properties.

Sorbitan monostearate: Derived from the berries of the mountain ash tree, sorbitan monostearate powder is a food-grade emulsifier and humectant used in natural lotions and creams.

Alginate: Derived from sea algae, sodium alginate powder is a water-soluble emulsifier and stabilizer that forms a colorless gel-like solution when mixed with liquids.

Isosteroyl lactylate: A derivative of lactic acid (a natural component of human skin,) isosteroyl lactylate is an alpha hydroxy acid which is an excellent humectant (water binding agent) that maintains the skin's pH level. It emulsifies and stabilizes oil in water.

Polysorbate 20: A food-grade emulsifier used to stabilize essential oils in aqueous solutions.

Modified lecithin: Originating from soybean oil, lecithin is a natural emulsifier and contains phospholipids, an integral part of all human and plant cells. Phospholipids from lecithin are remarkable emollients, moisturizers and cell-regenerating substances when added to skincare formulas.

Vitamin A: (Retinol) Vitamin A is available in oil form and is a valuable nourishing compound and skin cell regenerator.

Vitamin C: (Ascorbic acid) Water-soluble Vitamin C is a potent anti-oxidant, greatly reducing the damage done to the skin by free radicals.

Vitamin E: (Tocopherol) Vitamin E is an oil-soluble, deep-moisturizing vitamin with remarkable anti-oxidant properties.

Grapefruit seed extract: A natural preservative, grapefruit seed extract is a broad spectrum, non-toxic, anti-microbial product derived from the seeds, pulp and white membrane of grapefruit.

Germaben II: Germaben II is a combination of propyl- and methyl-paraben and diazolidinyl urea, a highly effective preservative that is considered safer than many other preservative systems.

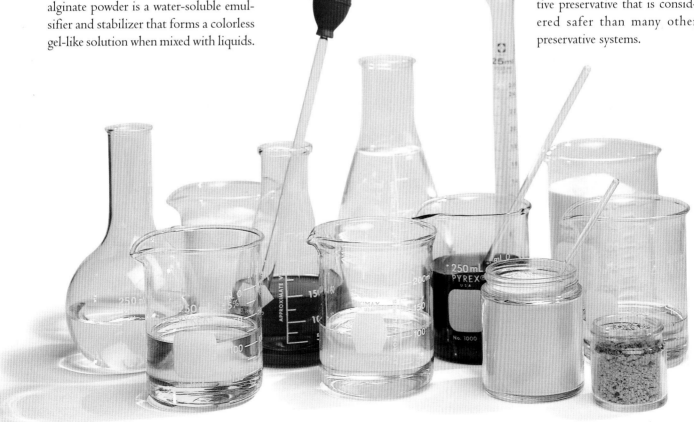

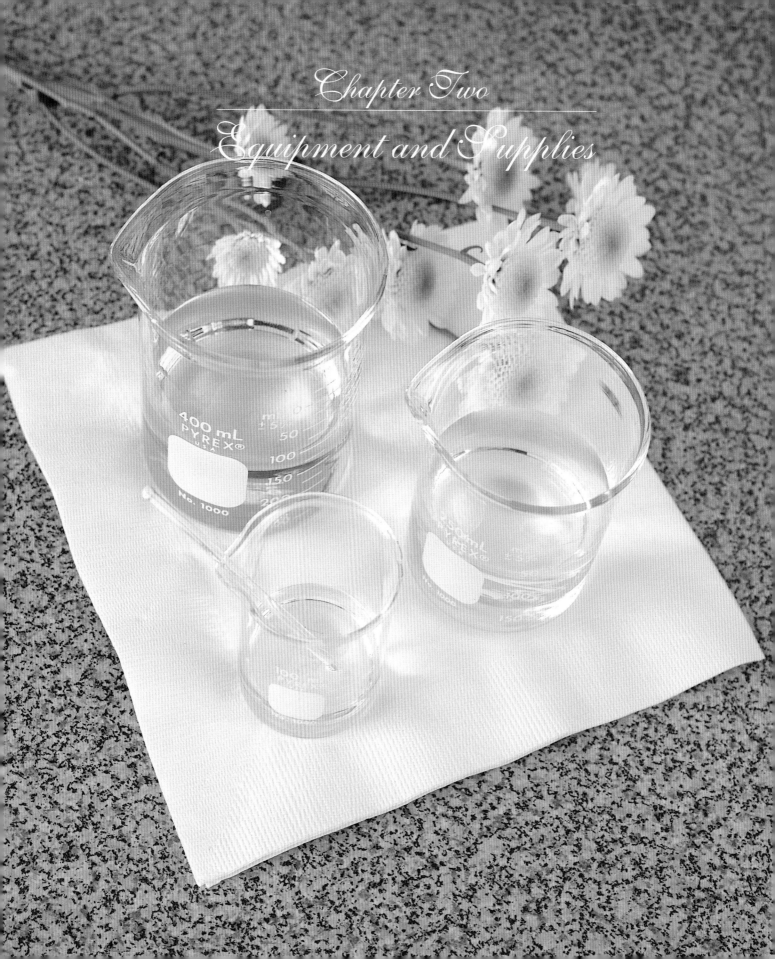

Equipment and Supplies

It's no coincidence that the kitchen has always been at the heart of the activity of creating natural bodycare preparations and home remedies. Known in earlier centuries as the 'stillroom,' the kitchen was the meeting place for the women of the house who took responsibility for harvesting, drying and storing herbs and botanicals and making the tinctures, tonics and salves that stocked the family medicine cupboard. Equipment used for preparing these homemade products has not changed much over the centuries. In fact, most of the equipment you will need to create the formulas on the following pages can be found right in your kitchen. If you are just starting to experiment with personal bodycare recipes, standard kitchen equipment and supplies will work very satisfactorily.

Should you decide that you will be making natural bodycare products on a regular basis, consider purchasing a separate set of kitchen equipment designated specifically for this purpose. Your new equipment need not be fancy or expensive. One critical consideration when making your own natural bodycare formulas is that the equipment be scrupulously clean (preferably sterilized before each use) so that your products ultimately have as long a shelf life as possible. By using this set of equipment for your cosmetic purposes only, you avoid the potential problems of contamination by food- or airborne bacteria which can lodge in cracks and crevices in glass and plastic containers which are used for other purposes. A small investment in your own personal equipment for making cosmetics at home will pay for itself within a few months, and is worthwhile when you consider the money you will save by making your own

fresh and natural cosmetic products.

Here is a complete range of the appliances, equipment and supplies you will need in order to create professional bodycare formulas at home:

DOUBLE BOILER OR 'BAIN-MARIE':

The classic way to heat waxes, oils and butters is in a 'bain-marie' or double boiler. These two-part metal pots are traditionally used to make cream sauces, gravies and other mixtures that need to be warmed slowly over indirect heat while being stirred by hand. With the advent of microwaves and packaged foods, double boilers are sometimes hard to find, but they are definitely worth the search. With a double boiler, the cosmetic ingredients stay within a workable temperature range, as the lower portion of the boiler transmits the heat to the upper container evenly and at temperatures never exceeding boiling point (212° F/100° C.) This is very important when you are working with volatile substances and materials such as beeswax, which has a flashpoint of 350° F/177° C. If you don't have a double boiler, select a heavy-bottomed stainless steel pot, half-fill it with boiling water, and use a glass bowl or jar to heat your cosmetic ingredients. Be careful to keep your stove burner at a low or medium setting, watch the inner container carefully to ensure that it doesn't tip over or break from the heat, and always use a heatproof mitt when handling the inner container.

NUT GRINDER OR COFFEE GRINDER:

A portable electric grinder will help you to prepare your own natural scrubs,

exfoliants and herbal mixes. Simply select the materials you wish to use and grind them to the consistency you want. Be sure to wipe the grinder out well afterwards. (Tip: cleaning out the grinder with a paper towel saturated with boiled water containing several drops of tea tree or thyme essential oil will keep the container clean and germ-free.)

SET OF GLASS MIXING BOWLS:

Sturdy clear glass mixing bowls are ideal for blending and mixing your customized natural creations and can be used for materials such as salts, grains, meals, powders and liquid emulsions. Glass is preferable to plastic or wood as it is hygienic, easily sterilized, and does not absorb or retain the odors or properties of the ingredients you are working with. Stainless steel (not aluminum) mixing bowls may also be used.

SET OF GLASS MEASURING CUPS WITH POUR SPOUTS

Clear glass measuring cups are perfect for measuring dry and liquid ingredients of all kinds. They can also be used as mixing containers for smaller amounts of liquids that can be blended with a wire whisk. Glass cups are preferable to plastic, as they can be sterilized in a dishwasher, and they do not absorb or retain oils or aromas. You may find that you like to work with cylindrical glass beakers, made of thinner glass that is marked with precise measurements in metric and imperial. Beakers are best suited for small mixtures containing finer materials, particularly when you are working with more expensive ingredients and want an extra degree of quality control. Laboratory-style beakers are easily obtained from scientific supply houses.

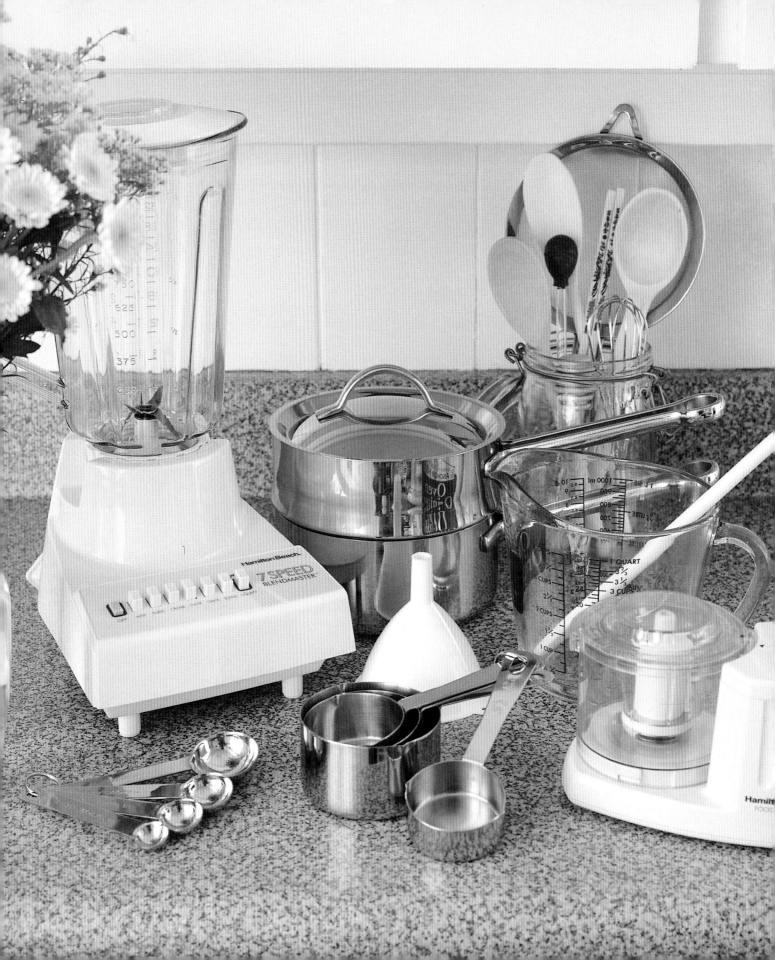

SET OF STAINLESS STEEL MEASURING SPOONS:

A set of kitchen spoons measuring from 1/4 tsp. up to 1 Tbsp. is an important aid in guaranteeing that you add the exact amounts of preservatives, vitamins and other special ingredients to your formulations for best results.

PLASTIC OR GLASS FUNNELS:

Several different sizes of funnels will enable you to easily decant your liquids, tonics, lotions, gels and oils into the finished bottles of your choice. Check the openings of the bottles you intend to use, and purchase funnels that rest firmly inside the opening. You can also modify the funnel to act as a sieve or strainer by using paperclips to attach filter papers, paper towels or cheesecloth across the bowl of the funnel so that liquids can gently filter through into the bottle beneath.

HARD PLASTIC OR WOODEN MIXING SPOONS:

Long-handled mixing spoons are useful for stirring and blending mixtures to a desired consistency. Non-porous hard plastic resists stains, cracks and bacteria. Working with spoons allows you to watch the stages of your formulas closely as you progress.

METAL WHISKS:

Large whisks are helpful for blending essential oils with dry materials such as salts and powders. Small whisks are useful for blending small amounts of wet and dry materials.

CHOPSTICKS, SPOONS AND STIRRING RODS:

Hard plastic chopsticks are excellent for thoroughly blending mixtures in measuring cups and beakers. Teaspoons are necessary for transferring creams and powders into small pots. Glass stirring rods are versatile and hygienic, and work well for mixing ingredients in small glass beakers and bowls.

DROPPERS AND PIPETTES:

Essential oil bottles usually come with integrated one-drop dispensers. Medicinal droppers (the kind with the rubber bulb) are a useful standby. Pipettes with calibrated stems are good for measuring large quantities of essential oils, and can be obtained from scientific supply houses. They can be flushed with alcohol to clean and sterilize them.

CANNING STYLE GLASS JELLY JARS WITH LIDS:

Clear glass jelly jars in various sizes (sold by the box in supermarkets) are invaluable for storing larger quantities of your completed products. Be sure to label and date your jars so that you keep a record of your creations and can check them periodically to ensure their freshness.

BOTTLES AND CONTAINERS:

Glass and plastic bottles with well-fitting lids are the best choice for your natural bodycare formulas. Glass bottles come in clear, frosted, amber (brown) and cobalt blue colors and are the bottles to choose if your recipes contain essential oils, salts, alcohol or carrier oils. Essential oil-based products are often packaged in colored glass bottles, which resist UV damage to the contents. European sizes of glass bottles usually run in 50 ml. increments. Plastic bottles with flip-top lids are very useful for gels and shampoos for use at home if you have children, have a concern about glass breakage, or if you need a lightweight, shatterproof package for travel. Opaque or white plastic is preferable. Standard sizes for most bottles are 2 oz., 4 oz. and 8 oz. Spray mister attachments can generally be purchased to fit most sizes of bottles. Wide-mouthed glass pots in small sizes up to 2 oz./60 ml. are useful for moisturizing creams, salves and solid perfumes.

OTHER USEFUL EQUIPMENT:

- stove top: gas or electric (for heating water and using the bain-marie)
- electric blender (for mixing lotions and creams at high speeds)
- kitchen scale (for working with dry ingredients)
- coffee maker (for making herbal infusions)
- filter papers and cheesecloth (for straining infusions and making face masks)
- electric juicer (for making fresh juices for facial treatments)
- strainers and sieves (for grain flours and herbal powders)
- ice cube tray (to make beeswax cubes, measure the size needed with a measuring spoon and water first; then spray an ice cube tray with vegetable cooking spray, pour melted beeswax and allow to cool: the beeswax cubes will pop right out!)
- decorative bottles, jars and corks (for storing your creations, or to give as gifts)

With this basic equipment at hand, you're ready to create healthy, natural cosmetics for yourself and your family and friends!

Chapter Three
Basic Techniques and Recipes

The first two chapters will have familiarized you with the natural ingredients and basic equipment needed to make natural bodycare formulas. If you have very little time to spare, you might want to purchase ready-made unfragranced bases to which you'll be adding pure essential oils, herbs and other ingredients. In this case, be sure to find a knowledgeable supplier or retailer who can assist you in selecting fragrance-free carrier bases made of natural ingredients. If you prefer to make your own unfragranced bases, this chapter will show you how. There are recipes on the following pages for mineral bath salts, dusting powder, bath oil, body oil, natural perfume, cleansing milk, body lotion, moisture cream, liquid soap, bath gel, shampoo and conditioner bases. As you become familiar with herbs and essential oils and start to make your own customized formulas for yourself, your friends and family, you'll be able to adjust the recipes to suit your particular needs.

Some of the recipes include herbs in their dried form, as well as herbal infusions and extracts. Ideally, if you have a small garden or windowbox, you can grow many herbs yourself and air-dry them in small bunches. If this is not possible, obtain your dried herbs from a specialist mail order supplier or local herb shop. Make sure that the herbs you purchase are fragrant and colorful. Herbs which are faded, brittle or odorless are old or have been exposed to sunlight, and their volatile plant oils have dispersed, greatly lessening their therapeutic value.

Herbal infusions are extremely easy to make. If you can make tea, you can make an infusion! Place 2 Tbsp. of your chosen loose dried herbs in a teapot, pour boiling distilled or spring water over them, stir them occasionally for 5 – 10 minutes, then leave the mixture to steep for a further 10 – 20 minutes. Pour the infusion through a fine mesh sieve or filter it through a cheesecloth-lined funnel into a glass kitchen jar. The longer the herbs are steeped, the stronger your infusion will be. The active botanical properties of the herbs are released into the water when infused. With cosmetic herbs such as those described on page 21, you can experiment with quantities and timing to make a fine, delicate infusion, or a robust, colorful and aromatic brew, depending on the recipe you are creating. When using herbal infusions in your recipes, substitute the exact amount of water called for in the recipe with the same amount of cooled herbal infusion.

Herbal extracts are made by preparing the dried herb with a solvent, typically alcohol, although vinegar and glycerin are sometimes used. Herbal extracts are called for in some recipes as they contain therapeutic organic acids, alkaloids and glucosides which are only available from the plant material when extracted with alcohol. To make an extract, place 2 Tbsp. of dried herbs into a wide-mouth glass jar and add 4 oz. of unflavored vodka and 4 oz. of distilled or spring water. Close the jar and keep it in a warm place for two weeks, shaking the jar daily. At the end of two weeks, strain or filter the extract into a clean glass bottle. Herbal extracts have a shelf life of many years, and add therapeutic and preservative properties to bodycare recipes. As you become familiar with the skin-healing herbs outlined in this book, you will enjoy making your own herbal infusions and extracts, knowing that you alone control the purity and effectiveness of your creations.

Infused oils are also easy to make and are an effective way of preserving the therapeutic qualities of specific herbs and botanicals in a mild, soothing natural oil base. Infused oil of calendula is a good example of an infused oil that has been used for centuries for skin and muscular conditions and to heal wounds and soften scar tissue. Natural perfumes can be made by infusing strong-scented flowers in oil (see page 97). To make an infused oil, pick flowers or herbs early in the morning, once the dew has dried and before the sun becomes too strong. Inspect the flowers and herbs carefully, and remove any wilted or damaged parts, insects or dirt. Layer the plant materials in a glass or ceramic container and pour golden olive oil over them ensuring that the plants are completely submerged. Place the covered container in a warm place like a windowsill or shelf away from direct sunlight, moisture or dust. Stir the contents frequently or gently shake the container each time you pass by. Continue this process for two weeks, making sure that the oil stays within a comfortable temperature range. After two weeks, gently filter the oil into dark glass bottles, discarding the plant solids. Cap and label the bottles, and store them in a cool, dark place.

Pure essential oils from plant sources are indispensable if you want to be able to make a wide variety of healthy, beautifying aromatherapy products. Please remember that in order to have a positive aromatherapeutic effect, your formulas should include only pure essential oils of botanical origin, and not aroma-chemical scents or 'fragrance oils.' The advantage of working with premium-quality pure essential oils is that they are naturally fragrant and they blend harmoniously with many different raw materials without a great deal of preparation. All pure essential oils display the clean, characteristic aroma of the plants from which they were obtained, and most people whose senses are not dulled from over-exposure to chemical scents will immediately and instinctively appreciate the difference. When used correctly and in the appropriate amounts, premium-quality pure essential oils will give your natural bodycare products a fragrant, healing quality that no commercial product can match.

Pure essential oils mix easily into carrier oils, lotions and gels, and need only be well stirred into the carrier base to blend them. In water-based solutions, they need an emulsifier, or will require a label bearing the old adage, "Shake well before using!" Dry materials such as salts, clays, starches, powdered milk, herbal powders and dried plant materials readily accept essential oils if they are gently blended together in a glass or ceramic bowl with a whisk or spoon. Some essential oils have antibacterial and preservative properties that extend the shelf life of products. When mixing full-strength essential oils into the carrier bases, use glass or ceramic containers whenever possible and avoid metal and plastic. Your completed product can be packaged in clear or colored glass or plastic containers.

The most useful essential oils to become familiar with for bodycare recipes are listed on page 23. There are currently about 100 pure essential oils, absolutes and oleoresins readily available in the marketplace. Select a reputable supplier and purchase premium-quality pure essential oils either by mail order or through one of the better natural foods, herb or specialty stores. If you find that you are drawn to working with these truly miraculous substances, read as much as you can about them, and take every opportunity to smell them firsthand. You will find that your nose is undoubtedly your best judge and guide as to their character, qualities and suitable uses in your products. Purchase a few good oils to begin an aromatic 'library' and experiment with blending drops of oils into small amounts of unfragranced bases to see how you like the consistency and aromatherapy results of your creations.

Many excellent books are available which describe pure essential oils in detail and give recommendations for their use in treating various conditions. Once you have acquired a few essential oils that capture your interest, you're ready to add them to the unfragranced carrier bases of your choice. If you wish to increase the aroma intensity of your recipes, carefully add more essential oil drop by drop until you have reached the desired fragrance and consistency, but be careful not to overdo it! Remember, with bodycare formulas, you want to achieve a soft, subtle natural aroma that will gently envelop the skin and bring healing qualities to the body and psyche, not a copy of the loud, overbearing scents associated with many mass-produced cosmetics. When combining essential oils with absolutes, bear in mind that absolutes are up to eight times stronger in aroma intensity than essential oils, so you will need to adjust your proportions accordingly, If you blend drop by drop, you will achieve the right result without overdoing it.

Creative blending is the most fascinating part of making your own natural cosmetics with pure essential oils and absolutes. With the advent of mind/body medicine, the relationship between physical and emotional states is now recognized, and creative blends address both. To make a harmonious blend or 'synergy', become familiar with the various families of essential oils – woody, spicy, floral, citrus, herbaceous. Generally, oils of one or two botanical families blend well together. Be innovative and experiment! Each essential oil has a special quality or 'note' (see page 23) which can be likened to music, mood or color. 'Top notes' are fresh, light and uplifting – the first impression. 'Middle notes' constitute the heart of the blend. 'Base notes' are rich, heavy and tenacious – they emerge slowly and linger awhile. In the practice of aromatherapy, top notes are considered to have a tonic, uplifting effect on the body/mind. Middle notes beneficially effect the major body systems including circulation and metabolism, and base notes are sedative, effectively relieving stress and tension. Each blend you make will be a personal, unique, alchemical formula! Once you have completed blending and making up your personalized creations, store them in UV-resistant glass and label and date them for future use.

Glossary of Cosmetic Terms

ABSOLUTES: Highly aromatic substances obtained from flowers too delicate for steam distillation by solvent extraction, absolutes retain the characteristic aroma of the flowers. Examples are rose absolute and jasmine absolute.

ALPHA HYDROXY ACIDS: Mild acidic compounds derived from various common fruits and vegetables, AHAs are a popular addition to creams and lotions for their light exfoliating and moisturizing effects.

ANTI-OXIDANTS: Naturally-occurring substances that have the ability to prevent peroxidation of natural oils, fats and food-grade materials by destructive free radicals, thus extending their healthy shelf life. Examples are Vitamins A, C and E.

BARRIER AGENTS: Substances having a large molecular structure that can create a film or deposit which, when applied, prevents external elements from affecting the skin. Examples are mineral oil and beeswax.

CARRIER OILS: Fresh vegetable, nut or seed oils act as 'carriers' when essential oils are added in up to 5% solution, allowing the oils to be easily applied to large areas of skin where they are absorbed. Examples are grapeseed oil and hazelnut oil.

COLD-PRESSED OILS: Natural oils that have been pressed from the plant material without heat, solvents or chemicals, retaining their original vitamins, minerals, amino acids and essential fatty acids. Examples are sweet almond oil and wheatgerm oil.

COLORING AGENTS: Substances used to color cosmetics, synthetically derived from coal tar (F, D & C colors and dyes), or natural colors from food grade sources. Examples of natural colors are chlorophyll, carotene, turmeric and beetroot powder.

EMOLLIENTS: Natural oils, fats and lipids that, when combined with water and other natural ingredients, form the basis for skin-nourishing natural cosmetic products. Examples are cold-pressed vegetable oils and plant butters.

EMULSIFIERS: Cosmetic ingredients which assist in combining oil, water and other ingredients in order to make a stable and homogenous emulsion (e.g. facial cream). Examples are polysorbate 20 and phospholipids (from lecithin.)

ESSENTIAL OILS: Volatile oils obtained from the leaves, roots, woods and flowers of various plants by steam distillation, each having the characteristic aroma and therapeutic qualities of the plant. Called 'essential' as they were originally believed to be essential to life and to contain the 'essence' of the plant. Examples are lavender and rosemary essential oils.

EXTRACTS: Solutions obtained by immersing fresh or dried herbs, woods, gums or resins in alcohol or an alcohol/water mixture to extract the beneficial properties from the plant material. Examples are tincture of benzoin and extract of yarrow herb.

HUMECTANTS: Substances that conserve the moisture content of lotions and creams, often by attracting moisture from the air. Examples are glycerin and floral waters.

INFUSED OILS: Steeping fresh or dried plant materials in a cold-pressed vegetable oil produces an infused oil which contains the therapeutic values of the plant material in an oily, emollient base. Examples are infused calendula oil and St. John's Wort oil.

LIPOSOMES: Microscopic hollow spherical structures composed of molecules that are small enough to penetrate the epidermis. It is believed that liposomes can enclose active ingredients, creating a 'delivery system' to bring ingredients deep within the skin's structure. Liposomes can be created in creams and lotions containing phospholipids when mixed at speeds exceeding 3,000 rpm in an electric blender.

PHOSPHOLIPIDS: Non-toxic, non-irritating skin moisturizers and repair compounds derived from soybean lecithin. Phospholipids are excellent emulsifiers and humectants which, when included in creams and lotions, greatly benefit dry, aging or damaged skin.

PRESERVATIVES: Bacteria and micro-organisms quickly multiply in fresh food-grade materials and spoil them. Preservatives inhibit the growth of bacteria and extend the useful life of cosmetics. Examples are Germaben II, grapefruit seed extract and certain essential oils.

SHELF LIFE: The amount of time a cosmetic can be kept at normal room temperature before being adversely affected by bacteria, peroxidation and chemical changes.

SURFACTANTS: 'Surface active agents' or surfactants are composed of compounds which, when combined with water, exhibit a foaming and cleansing action on the skin. Examples are liquid soap bases and polyglucose, derived from sugars and fatty acids.

UNFRAGRANCED BASES: Combinations of dry or liquid natural ingredients that are prepared without the addition of natural or synthetic fragrances. Unfragranced bases may be customized into healthful body cosmetics through the addition of naturally aromatic pure essential oils of botanic origin.

TABLE OF EQUIVALENTS AND CONVERSIONS
U.S. - METRIC FLUID VOLUME

	TEA-SPOONS	TABLE-SPOONS	FLUID OUNCES	1/4 CUP	1/2 CUP	1 CUP	*MILLI-LITERS
1 TEA-SPOON	1	1/3	1/6	1/12	1/24	1/48	5
1 TABLE-SPOON	3	1	1/2	1/4	1/8	1/16	15
1 FLUID OUNCE	6	2	1	1/2	1/4	1/8	30
1/4 CUP	12	4	2	1	1/2	1/4	60
1/2 CUP	24	8	4	2	1	1/2	120
1 CUP	48	16	8	4	2	1	240
1 MILLI-LITER	0.203 OR 1/5	0.068	0.34	0.017	0.008	0.004	1

*All amounts are rounded off

True aromatherapy recipes include pure essential oils (PEOs) which are measured in drops and milliliters

There are approximately = 100 drops = 5 ml. = 1 tsp.

Throughout this book, pure essential oils are referred to in the recipes with the designation 'PEO'

MEASUREMENT GUIDELINES

The aroma intensity of pure essential oils varies from oil to oil, and often from batch to batch. Ingredients in different unfragranced carrier bases likewise vary, so the aroma intensity and texture of your finished products will display slightly different characteristics each time. Add oils carefully drop by drop, mixing thoroughly, and do not exceed these guidelines. 'Drops' refers to drops from an integrated drop dispenser of an essential oil bottle. Bear in mind that absolutes are up to eight times stronger in aroma intensity than essential oils, so adjust your measurements accordingly. Here are some guidelines:

Bath Salts: Add 10 - 15 drops of essential oil/s to each 2 oz. (1/4 cup) unfragranced bath salts.

Dusting Powders: Add 10 - 15 drops of essential oil/s to each 4 oz. (1/2 cup) unfragranced powder base.

Body Oils: Add 20 - 25 drops of essential oil/s to each 1 oz. (30 ml.) unfragranced carrier oil/s.

Bath Oils: Add 20 - 25 drops of essential oil/s to each 1 oz. (30 ml.) unfragranced carrier oil/s.

Body Lotions: Add 20 - 25 drops of essential oil/s to each 1 oz. (30 ml.) unfragranced lotion.

Cleansing Milks: Add 10 - 15 drops of essential oil/s to each 1 oz. (30 ml.) unfragranced cleansing emulsion base.

Facial Oils and Creams: Add 5 - 10 drops of essential oil/s to each 1 oz. (30 ml.) unfragranced oil or cream.

Bath and Shower Gels: Add 10 - 15 drops of essential oil/s to each 1 oz. (30 ml.) unfragranced bath or shower gel base.

Liquid Soap Cleansers: Add 10 - 15 drops of essential oil/s to each 1 oz. (30 ml.) unfragranced liquid soap base.

Hair Shampoo: Add 10 - 15 drops of essential oil/s to each 1 oz. (30 ml.) unfragranced shampoo base.

Hair Conditioner: Add 10 - 15 drops of essential oil/s to each 1 oz. (30 ml.) unfragranced conditioner base.

Mineral Bath Salts and Dusting Powders

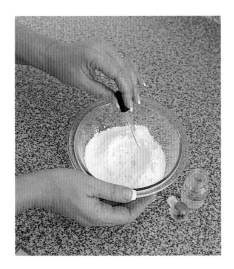

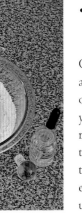

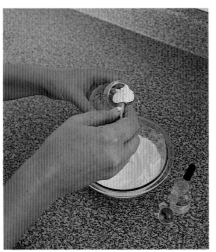

MINERAL BATH SALTS

These snowy-white bath salts contain a high percentage of natural minerals and trace elements which, when added to bathwater, create a soothing and detoxifying personal spa experience. Select sea salts that have been naturally dried and packaged without the addition of bleaching or anti-caking chemicals. Dead Sea mineral salts provide therapeutic elements to aid in the improvement of skin conditions, while Epsom salts relieve pain or inflammation in muscles and joints.

- *1 cup (8 oz.) coarse sea salts*
- *1/2 cup (4 oz.) fine sea salts*
- *1/4 cup (2 oz) Dead Sea mineral salts*
- *1/4 cup (2 oz.) Epsom salts (magnesium sulfate)*

Combine the salts in a large glass bowl, and stir them well with a wooden spoon or wire whisk. Add the essential oils of your choice drop by drop until you have reached the desired consistency and intensity of fragrance. To add a subtle shine to the salts, drizzle a little vegetable glycerin or sweet almond oil over them. Stir until the salts are completely blended, and store them in airtight glass containers.

Uncolored natural bath salts last longer than colored salts, but if you want to color them, you have some options. Natural plant-, herb- and mineral-derived powders will add subtle color to salts. Experiment with the following ingredients to achieve a range of natural colors: chlorophyll, barley or wheatgrass powder (green); spirulina or sea-blue algae (blue-green); turmeric (yellow); paprika (orange); beetroot powder (rose pink) or herbal powders such as benzoin, myrrh, frankincense or sandalwood (sandy beige).

DUSTING POWDER

Natural dusting powders contain a variety of combinations of food-grade starches, powders and clays, omitting powdered minerals such as talc that can cause respiratory problems. Dry clay powders have a crisp feel and deodorant and absorbent qualities, while fine-milled flours and starches lend a satiny feel and soft finish to powders. Familiarize yourself with the various available food-grade powders and clays by rubbing them between your fingertips to assess the degree of 'slip' you like. Here is a basic recipe for an unfragranced body powder:

- *1 cup (8oz.) cornstarch*
- *1/4 cup (2 oz.) arrowroot powder*
- *2 Tbsp. white clay powder*
- *2 Tbsp. baking soda (sodium bicarbonate)*

Carefully measure the powders into a glass bowl, stirring slowly with a wire whisk. Add essential oils to the powder mix drop by drop, ensuring that the drops are broken up in the powder as you go. Continue to stir the powder in concentric circles until the entire mixture gives off the desired aroma intensity. Let the powder sit for 10 – 20 minutes, stir with the whisk, and add more essential oils if desired. Once you have achieved the desired aroma and consistency, spoon the powder into small shaker-type glass or plastic jars. Salt and pepper shakers, grated cheese dispensers and small flour sifters make excellent containers for body powders, foot powders and dry shampoos. Cap your containers well, label them and keep them away from sunlight, heat or excessive moisture. Use as needed.

Oils and Perfumes

BATH OIL

To make a silky, fine-textured bath oil, select a light cold-pressed oil and add a percentage of modified lecithin, which will act as an emulsifier, dispersing the oil through the water and reducing the tendency of the oil to cling to the tub.

- *8 oz. (240 ml.) cold-pressed oil such as sesame or sweet almond*
- *1 Tbsp.(15 ml.) modified lecithin*
- *1 Tbsp. (15 ml.) vegetable glycerin*

Combine the ingredients in a glass bowl, stirring together well. You now have a premium-quality, unfragranced bath oil base to which you can add your favorite essential oil or blend of essential oils. As a standard rule of thumb, add 20 – 25 drops of essential oil to each ounce of bath oil. Continue stirring until the oil is smooth and fragrant. Pour the oil through a funnel into a glass or plastic bottle and cap tightly.

BODY OIL

A multi-purpose oil for massage, skincare, or for use after a bath or shower, this basic bodycare recipe combines cold-pressed vegetable and nut oils with skin-nurturing specialty oils and vitamins.

- *4 oz. (120 ml.) hazelnut oil*
- *4 oz. (120 ml.) pecan or safflower oil*
- *1/2 oz. (15 ml.) wheatgerm oil*
- *1 tsp. (5 ml.) Vitamin E*

Combine the natural oils and Vitamin E in a bowl, and stir until blended. Pour the oil through a funnel into a bottle and cap tightly. You can add up to 200 drops of the essential oils or oil blend of your choice to 8 oz./240 ml. of carrier oil.

NATURAL PERFUME

Natural perfumes combine fragrant oils and exotic absolutes in a base of refined jojoba oil or alcohol. Experimenting with the quantities of absolutes or essential oils will reveal your preferences for aroma intensity, concentration and favored perfume base. Don't forget, when creating a well-balanced composition containing top, middle and base notes, that absolutes are much more intense than essential oils in fragrance level.

- *1 oz. (30 ml.) refined jojoba oil (or 90-proof unflavored vodka)*
- *20 drops absolute (or 50 drops essential oil or blend)*

Stir the absolute or essential oil blend into the jojoba oil or vodka until well blended and pour through a funnel into a decorative perfume bottle with airtight stopper. Apply as needed.

SOLID PERFUME

In a bain-marie or in a glass measuring cup inside a pot of boiling water, melt:

- *1 tsp. beeswax*
- *2 Tbsp. (30 ml.) cold-pressed oil*

Once the mixture is melted, stir it thoroughly and leave it to cool. Before it turns opaque, add 20 drops absolute or 50 drops of essential oil or blend and stir well. Pour the mixture into a glass jar and leave it to cool. It will solidify in the jar.

To make a natural lip balm, substitute shea butter or cocoa butter for the beeswax in the recipe above. Add a few pinches of carnauba or candelilla wax for gloss and shine and citrus or mint essential oils for flavor and aroma.

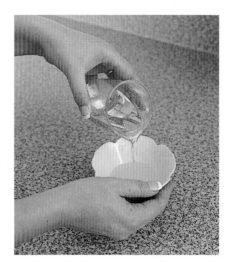
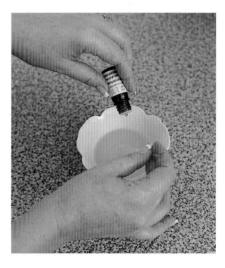
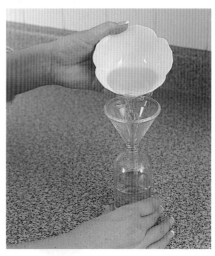

Lotions and Creams

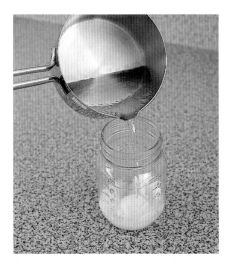

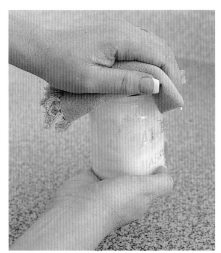

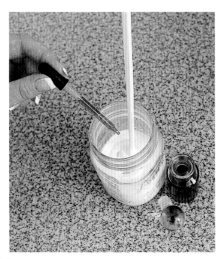

BODY LOTION

A nourishing natural body lotion is simple to make with this one-jar process.

- *2 Tbsp. (30 ml.) cold-pressed oil*
- *2 Tbsp. shea butter or cocoa butter*
- *2 Tbsp. sorbitan monostearate*
- *2 tsp. (10 ml.) isosteroyl lactylate*
- *1/2 tsp. Vitamin E*
- *1/2 tsp. modified lecithin*

Place the ingredients in a durable 8 oz. (240 ml.) glass kitchen jar. Bring 6 oz. (180 ml.) distilled or spring water or herbal infusion to a boil, and pour it over the ingredients. Cap tightly, cover the jar with a folded handtowel and shake the jar for 30 seconds. Uncap the jar and leave the lotion to cool for about 30 minutes. Add 20 drops of lemon juice. To preserve the lotion, stir in 1/2 tsp. grapefruit seed extract or 1/2 tsp. Germaben II while the lotion is cooling. Cap the bottle and shake again, then leave it to set up to a thick, smooth consistency.

MOISTURE CREAM

To make a rich, nourishing cream base, simply adapt the above recipe as follows:

- *increase the cold-pressed oil to 3 Tbsp. (45 ml.)*
- *increase the sorbitan monostearate to 3 Tbsp.*
- *decrease the amount of the boiled water or herbal infusion to 4 oz. (120 ml.)*

Follow the instructions for 'Body Lotion' above. The cream will have the consistency of a thin lotion until cooled. Add the lemon juice and preservatives while the mixture is cooling. Pour into several cream jars, cover them and let them cool overnight in a warm dry place. The cream will solidify overnight and gain a rich, smooth texture.

LIPOSOME BODY LOTION

Place 8 oz. (240 ml.) distilled water or herbal infusion in a blender with 1/2 tsp. grapefruit seed extract (or Germaben II.) Add 1 tsp. alginate powder and blend for 15 seconds. Add 30 drops of lemon juice. In a glass jar, mix the following:

- *2 tsp. (10 ml.) cold-pressed oil*
- *2 tsp. (10 ml.) modified lecithin*
- *2 tsp. (10 ml.) isosteroyl lactylate*
- *1/2 tsp. Vitamin E*

Pour the contents of the glass jar over the blender contents and blend the mixture for 45 seconds to form liposomes. Pour the lotion through a funnel into a clean bottle and cap tightly

CLEANSING MILK

A gentle cleansing milk that removes make-up, even eye make-up, while deep cleansing and softening the skin. Mix 2 oz. (60 ml.) polyglucose with 3 oz. (90 ml.) of distilled water or herbal infusion in a 8 oz. (240 ml.) glass jar. Then, mix the following oil-soluble ingredients in a second jar:

- *4 oz. (120 ml.) cold-pressed oil*
- *2 Tbsp. sorbitan monostearate powder*
- *1 tsp. (5 ml.) isosteroyl lactylate*

Place both uncapped jars in a pot half-full of hot water on the stovetop and heat the jars very gently until both ingredients register 140° F/60° C when measured with a thermometer, and all ingredients are dissolved. Combine the ingredients in one jar, cap tightly, cover with a folded handtowel, and shake the jar for 30 seconds. Let the mixture cool and add 1/2 tsp. preservative of your choice. Pour through a funnel into a bottle.

Cleansers and Haircare

BATH AND SHOWER GEL

A multi-purpose bath and shower gel made with mild and gentle cleansing agents.

- *4 oz. (120 ml.) distilled water or herbal infusion*
- *2 oz. (60 ml.) polyglucose*
- *1 oz. (30 ml.) coco betaine*
- *1 tsp. xanthan gum*
- *1 tsp. (5 ml.) modified lecithin*
- *1/2 tsp. grapefruit seed extract or Germaben II*

Combine all the ingredients in a blender, adding the xanthan gum powder last. Run blender on the lowest setting for 5-10 seconds, The mixture will be white and frothy. Pour the liquid through a funnel into a clean bottle and cap tightly.

LIQUID SOAP CLEANSER

A mild and effective cleanser for those who prefer a soap to a lotion cleanser.

- *1 cup (8 oz.) liquid coconut soap**
- *2 cups (16 oz.) distilled water or herbal infusion*
- *2 Tbsp. (30 ml.) modified lecithin*
- *2 Tbsp. (30 ml.) cold-pressed oil*
- *2 tsp. (10 ml.) grapefruit seed extract or Germaben II*

*You may substitute any good quality, unfragranced vegetable-based soap or soap flakes for the liquid coconut soap.

Using a bain-marie or glass bowl placed inside a pot of boiling water, heat the ingredients gently, stirring with a spoon or whisk. Once the soap, lecithin and oil are completely dissolved, allow to cool, and store the liquid mixture in a glass jar for future use.

HAIR SHAMPOO

A gentle hair shampoo for everyday use. Herbal infusions add to the effectiveness of the shampoo. For all hair types.

- *4 oz. (120 ml.) polyglucose*
- *2 oz. (60 ml.) coco betaine*
- *2 oz. (60 ml.) distilled water or herbal infusion*
- *1 tsp. (5 ml.) sucrose cocoate*
- *1 tsp. (5 ml.) isosteroyl lactylate*
- *1/2 tsp. modified lecithin*
- *1/2 tsp. grapefruit seed extract or Germaben II*

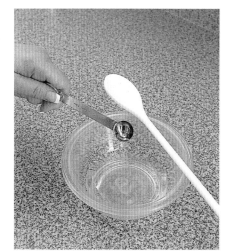

Mix all ingredients except the coco betaine together in a glass bowl and stir slowly with a spoon or whisk. Add the betaine slowly and continue to mix until the liquid becomes thicker. Pour through a funnel into a clean bottle and cap tightly.

HAIR CONDITIONER

Place 8 oz. (240 ml.) distilled or spring water or herbal infusion in a blender with 1/2 tsp. grapefruit seed extract or Germaben II. Add I tsp. alginate powder and blend for one minute. Add 30 drops of lemon juice. Then place the following ingredients in a glass bowl:

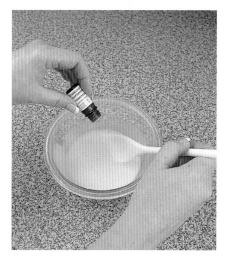

- *1 Tbsp. (15 ml.) cold-pressed oil*
- *1 tsp. (5 ml.) polyglucose*
- *1 tsp. (5 ml.) coco betaine*
- *1 tsp. (5 ml.) isosteroyl lactylate*
- *1/2 tsp. modified lecithin*
- *1/2 tsp. grapefruit seed extract or Germaben II*

Pour the ingredients from the blender gently over the ingredients in the bowl, stirring slowly. When the ingredients are well blended, pour through a funnel into a clean bottle and cap tightly.

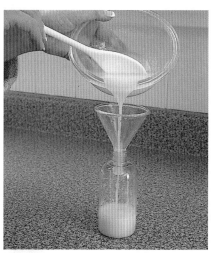

Chapter Four
Natural Haircare

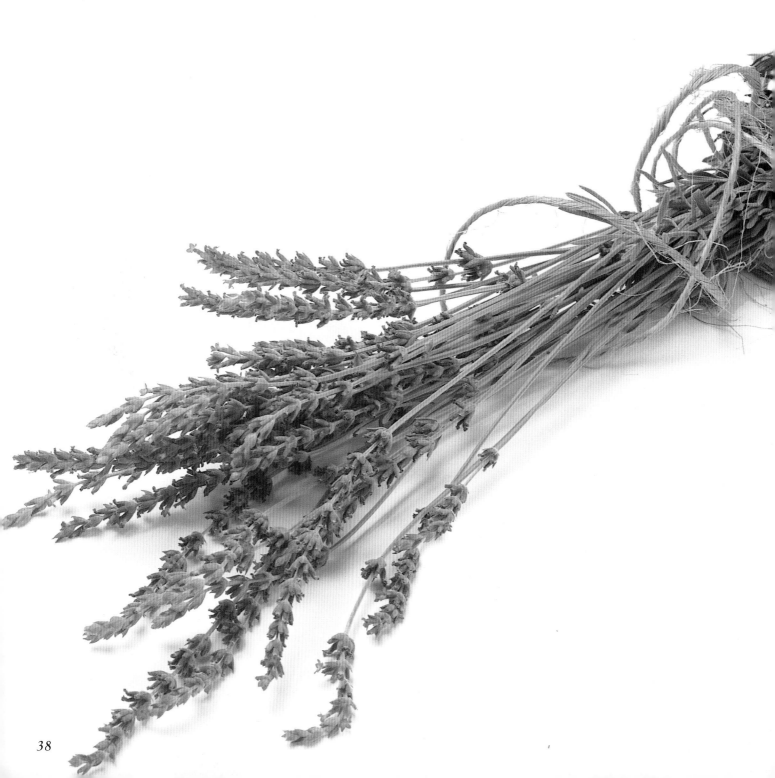

Introduction to Natural Haircare

The subject of hair — its care, maintenance, design and adornment — has held a certain fascination for people for centuries. Hair, like makeup and clothing, is an accurate barometer of the political, social and economic condition of cultures through history. Our perception of ourselves — our youthfulness, self-esteem and well-being — is often determined by the health and appearance of our hair. We even describe a day when everything is going wrong as a 'bad hair day!' Very few of us are happy with our hair in its natural state. We cut it, shave it, bleach and color it, straighten, wave and curl it, and subject it to a string of chemical and mechanical abuses to follow fashion and our own perception of beauty and style. None of this constitutes 'natural' treatment of the hair, but it makes us feel good about ourselves and how we present ourselves to the outside world. If your hair is going to be undergoing treatments with chemicals on a regular basis, it makes sense to ensure that it is as healthy as possible in its natural state. Simple shampoos, conditioners, scalp toners and hot oil treatments, diet, supplementation, regular brushing and massage are the best ways to ensure that your scalp and hair are in peak condition.

Hair has an intriguing, complex structure that originates deep within the dermis of the scalp. The average human head contains over 100,000 hairs growing at a rate of 1/10th of an inch in one month. Hair has an integral 'growth phase' of five years of more, interspersed with a 'rest phase' of approximately three months. Each hair shaft is made of three parts: the cuticle, cortex and medulla. The medulla constitutes the central 'core' of the hair. The cortex, composed of minute strands called 'fibrils,' forms about 80% of the hair, which is mainly made of keratin, a protein. The cuticle or outer layer of the hair has five to ten layers of overlapping colorless scales which protect the cortex. These scales can be easily damaged by excess shampooing and chemical treatments, heat, over-handling, sun and environmental influences. Care of the scalp is important too, as it is the health of the scalp that largely determines the appearance and longevity of the hair. Healthy hair originates in healthy follicles that ideally are nourished by a rich network of blood capillaries delivering nutrients and vitamins to the roots of the hair. If circulation is poor due to tight muscles from stress and tension, inadequate diet, lack of massage and use of follicle-clogging hair products, the hair will be sparse, weak and easily damaged.

Technically, while the scalp is a living organism, hair is not — it is composed of keratinized proteins which do not contain living cells. Sebaceous glands at the scalp's surface provide sebum, which lubricates the hair shaft, but only for the first inch or two of its length. In order to stimulate and condition the hair shaft, resulting in thick, resilient hair, scalp massage and nourishment of the scalp through tonics and hot oil treatments are two key necessities. Proper scalp massage dramatically improves the health and appearance of normal hair, and has often been demonstrated to make radical and positive changes in the appearance of thinning and receding hair. To perform an effective scalp massage, bend forward from the waist until your head is below heart level. Using the fingertips of both hands, push against the head as if you were holding a large ball. With firm, small, circular motions, rotate your fingertips around your scalp. Do not use superficial friction motions which will only stress or break the hair at the scalp surface. Then, with your head upright, push your fingertips up your neck and past the front of your ears, assisting the blood flow to the scalp, and finish by gently fanning your fingers through your hair. This simple but important activity will work wonders for the overall condition of your hair and scalp.

You can also further help the health of your hair by acquiring a natural bristle brush with rounded tips (the kind with the bristles embedded in a rubber pneumatic cushion is best) as well as a blunt-toothed wooden or thick plastic comb. Brush and use the massage technique frequently, especially whenever you use the scalp tonics, hot oil treatments and other natural haircare formulas in this chapter. All the recipes on the following pages have been designed to improve the condition of your hair and scalp naturally using safe and effective botanical ingredients. The shampoos are formulated with mild, low-sudsing cleansers and therapeutic essential oils. The tonics will refresh, cleanse and energize the scalp. Finally, the deep conditioners will nourish the hair roots and bring body and sheen to your hair. These treatments will also prove helpful if you color or perm your hair. A natural haircare program will improve the health of the hair and make it more resistant to the various challenges that affect it on a daily basis. After just a few weeks using massage and natural hair treatments, you will see positive changes in the health and appearance of your 'crowning glory'.

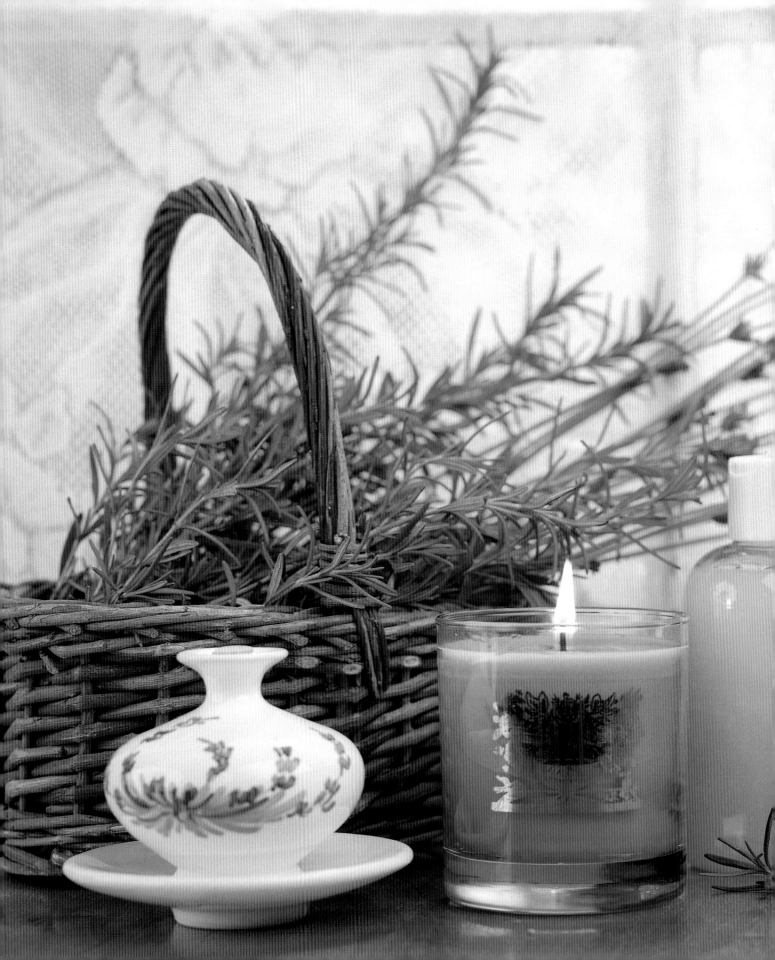

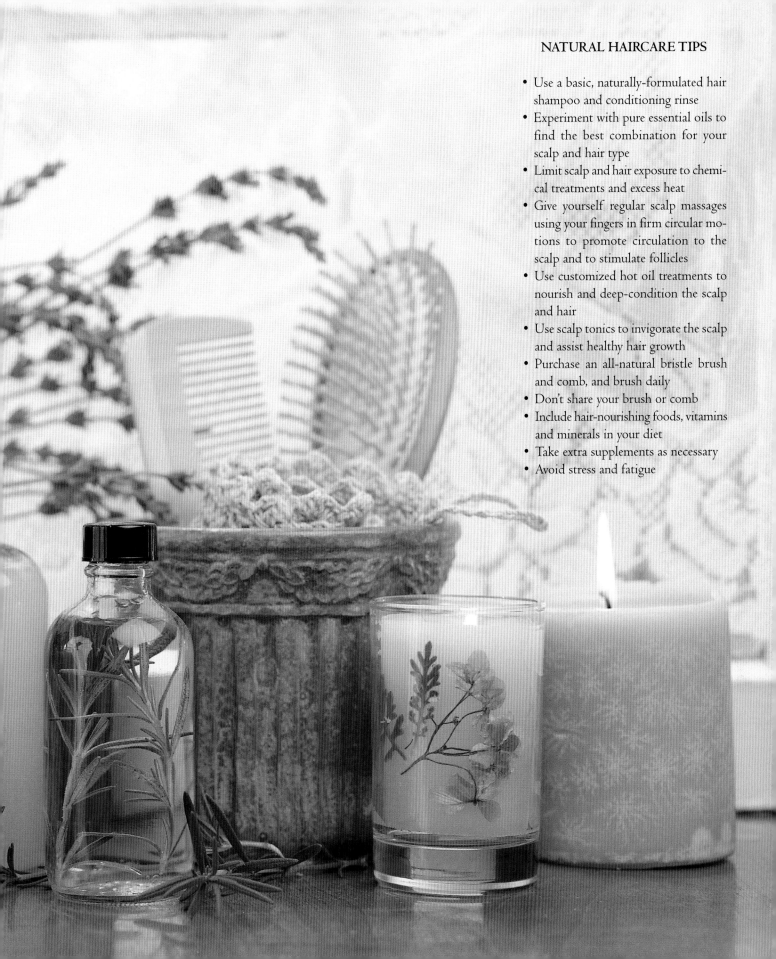

NATURAL HAIRCARE TIPS

- Use a basic, naturally-formulated hair shampoo and conditioning rinse
- Experiment with pure essential oils to find the best combination for your scalp and hair type
- Limit scalp and hair exposure to chemical treatments and excess heat
- Give yourself regular scalp massages using your fingers in firm circular motions to promote circulation to the scalp and to stimulate follicles
- Use customized hot oil treatments to nourish and deep-condition the scalp and hair
- Use scalp tonics to invigorate the scalp and assist healthy hair growth
- Purchase an all-natural bristle brush and comb, and brush daily
- Don't share your brush or comb
- Include hair-nourishing foods, vitamins and minerals in your diet
- Take extra supplements as necessary
- Avoid stress and fatigue

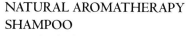

Natural Shampoos

The purpose of a natural shampoo is to thoroughly cleanse the hair and scalp without stripping them of their protective oils. Many of the cheaper commercial shampoos use harsh surfactants as a base, which can disrupt the natural growth cycle of the hair, either by over-drying the scalp through too-frequent use or by depositing a waxy layer that clogs the follicles and affects healthy hair growth. Synthetic fragrances and other chemical ingredients in the formula can also cause problems. A shampoo by definition contains the same type of cleansing surfactants as do soaps, so the key in a natural product is to use cleansers which are mild and non-irritating, such as polyglucoside or sucrose cocoate, derived from glucose (sugar) and fatty acids. Oilier hair will benefit from a modified cleanser based on liquid coconut soap with humectants such as lecithin and honey. Over-washing of the hair is a common problem which leads to scalp dryness, over- and under-active sebum production and hair that is lack-luster, brittle or malnourished. A classic

European 'dry shampoo' recipe is given which will be very helpful if you travel frequently or would like to experiment with cleansing your hair without constantly exposing it to tap water, chemicals and detergents. Lavender and rosemary essential oils provide the clean, fresh herbaceous aroma in these shampoos.

NATURAL HERBAL SHAMPOO FOR OILY HAIR

This low-sudsing scalp and hair cleanser will remove excess oil, regulate scalp function, and leave the hair clean.

- *5 oz. (150 ml.) unfragranced liquid soap*
- *2 oz. (60 ml.) aloe vera gel*
- *1 oz. (30 ml.) nettle extract*
- *1 Tbsp. (15 ml.) lemon juice*
- *1 tsp. (5 ml.) unpasteurized honey*
- *1 tsp. (5 ml.) modified lecithin*
- *30 drops rosemary PEO*
- *30 drops lavender PEO*

Combine all ingredients, stir until well blended, and pour into a bottle. Use as needed.

NATURAL AROMATHERAPY SHAMPOO

A gentle, fresh-smelling shampoo which effectively cleanses scalp and hair without disrupting their natural functions. For all hair types, especially normal to dry.

- *8 oz. (240 ml.) unfragranced shampoo base (see Chapter Three)*
- *30 drops rosemary PEO*
- *30 drops lavender PEO*

Pour the unfragranced shampoo base into a measuring cup or beaker, and stir in the essential oils. When the mixture is fully blended, pour through a funnel into a plastic squeeze bottle. Use as often as needed.

CLASSIC EUROPEAN DRY SHAMPOO

A lifesaver when travelling, camping, or when you simply do not have enough time to wash and style your hair. White clay absorbs excess oil, dirt and sebum while essential oils refresh and cleanse. For all hair types.

- *4 Tbsp. white clay powder*
- *1 Tbsp. cornstarch*
- *15 drops rosemary PEO*
- *15 drops lavender PEO*

Mix the dry materials in a bowl and, using a small whisk, blend in the essential oils drop by drop. Spoon the powder through a funnel into a small plastic squeeze bottle. To use the shampoo, part the hair in sections and dab small amounts of the powder onto the scalp with a cotton ball. Wait a minute or two, then brush well with a natural bristle hairbrush.

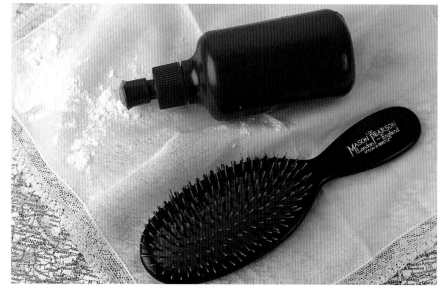

Natural Conditioners

Conditioning your hair after shampooing is important if you have dry, brittle hair or if you frequently color, bleach or chemically treat your hair. If your hair and scalp are naturally healthy and you are following the recommended steps for optimizing your hair's health with massage, hot oil treatments and scalp toners, you will enjoy using the light conditioning rinses described here. Cheaper commercial shampoos are made with strong surfactant bases that cause the pH of the hair to become excessively alkaline after shampooing. This disturbs the hair cuticle, roughening the shaft so that the hair becomes brittle and dull, breaking easily and lacking a natural sheen. Many commercial conditioners contain waxes, polymers or cellulose compounds which coat the hair shaft, creating a buildup which must be removed by the use of these detergent shampoos, resulting in an unsatisfactory cycle in which the hair is alternately stripped of natural oils and coated with heavier synthetic ones. If you have been unable to find a commercial conditioner suited to your particular hair type, try these simple, natural alternatives. For intensive conditioning, use hair repair complexes which include natural oils and vitamins in their formulation. Once every 4 – 6 weeks, apply a nutritious botanical hair pack if your hair is really dry or damaged. The recipes below provide you with choices for natural conditioning and management of your hair.

CONDITIONING ROSEMARY VINEGAR FOR HAIR

Mix equal parts of apple cider vinegar and water together in a glass, and stir in 10 drops of rosemary oil. Gently pour over washed hair, working in with fingertips, wait a few minutes, rinse out and towel dry. The vinegar smell vanishes as the hair dries. Your hair will be smooth and shiny with a fresh, herbal fragrance.

BEER RINSE WITH PATCHOULI

Stir 6 drops of patchouli oil into a glass of beer (flat beer is fine.) Gently pour over washed hair, working in with fingertips, wait a few minutes, rinse out and towel dry. Beer gives the hair body and sheen, and the patchouli oil conditions and fragrances.

NATURAL AROMATHERAPY CONDITIONER

A basic natural conditioner with added pure essential oils to provide aromatherapeutic benefits. For all hair types.

- *8 oz. (240 ml.) unfragranced hair conditioner base (see Chapter Three)*
- *30 drops rosemary PEO*
- *30 drops lavender PEO*

Stir the essential oils into the unfragranced hair conditioner base in a measuring cup or beaker until well blended. Pour through a funnel into a plastic squeeze bottle. To use, gently squeeze water from the hair, apply the conditioner, wait 1 – 3 minutes depending on the amount of conditioning needed, rinse and towel dry hair.

INTENSIVE BOTANICAL HAIR MASK

An intensive nutrient pack to provide damaged hair with body and luster. Use every 4 – 6 weeks for healthy, shiny hair.

- *2 oz. (60 ml.) almond oil*
- *1 oz. (30 ml.) avocado oil*
- *1/2 avocado*
- *juice of 1/2 lemon*
- *1 egg*
- *1/2 tsp. Vitamin E*
- *30 drops sweet orange PEO*

Mash the avocado and blend it with the rest of the ingredients in a bowl until smooth. Dampen your hair with warm water and towel dry. Apply the mask mixture liberally to your hair, massaging into the ends, and leave on for 15 – 20 minutes before rinsing off first with warm, then hot water. Shampoo lightly, dry and style naturally. Your hair will feel thick and healthy, with a smooth texture and beautiful shine.

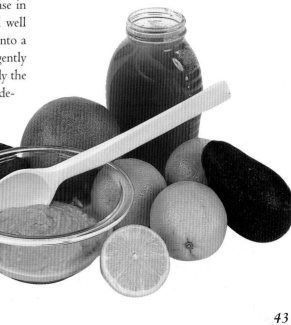

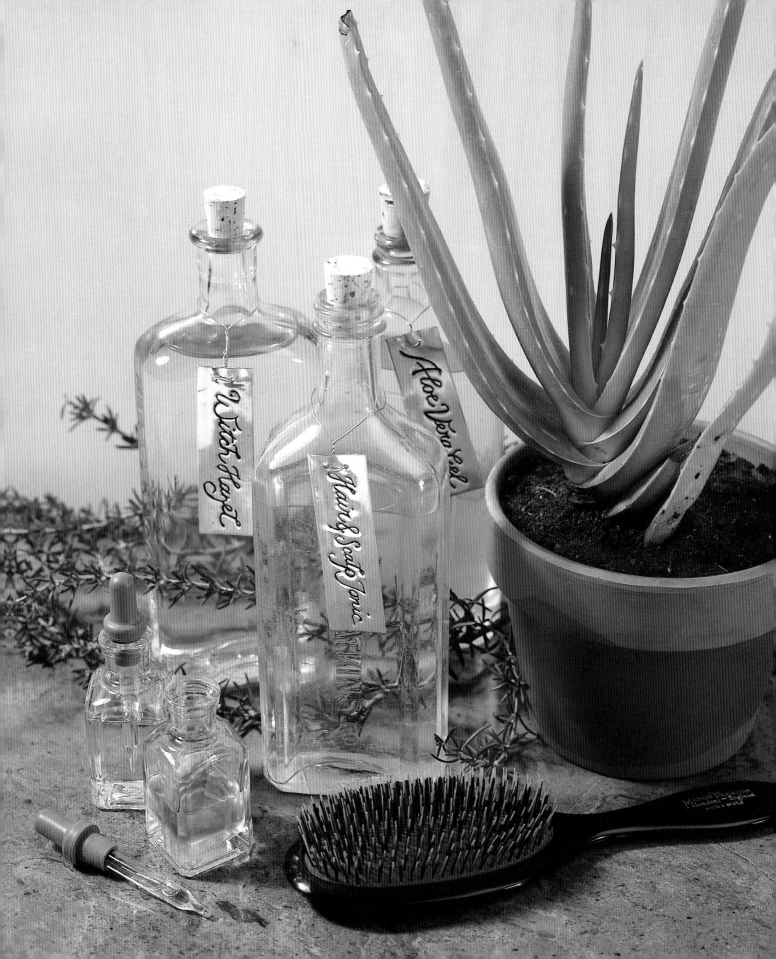

Aromatic Vinegars & Tonics

Scalp tonics and aromatic vinegars are a wonderful natural way to cleanse your scalp, banish headaches and muscle tension and clear your mind at the same time. Invigorating scalp tonics, mostly alcohol- and water-based, were a mainstay in our grandparents' time. Interestingly enough, many of our forebears boasted full heads of healthy hair well into their later years through the use of these simple but highly effective aromatic tonics. Many of the tonics also contained herbal extracts and essences that kept the hair youthful, thick and lustrous, with a minimum of gray. Scalp tonics are important for two reasons: first, they are the perfect medium for incorporating into a holistic scalp massage program; and second, they prevent the clogging of hair follicles by commercial hair product deposits, resulting in healthier, stronger hair. Pure essential oils make great additions to scalp tonics, as do vitamins and botanical extracts. The volatile base of the tonic stimulates the hair follicles and delivers essential oils and nutrients directly to the hair roots. Scalp massage using the pads of the fingertips in firm circular motions loosens the galea (the broad muscle which runs over the top of the scalp) and prepares the entire scalp to receive the nutrients. The deep, consistent movements of the massage also provide blood circulation to the scalp and stimulate hair growth.

SCALP TONIC FOR THINNING HAIR

This brisk and invigorating vitamin tonic is designed to be applied once or twice daily to activate previously-clogged hair follicles. The addition of vitamins A, B, C and E is optional, but is recommended if you wish to stimulate hair growth. For all hair types.

- 2 oz. (60 ml.) distilled or spring water
- 2 oz. (60 ml.) unflavored vodka
- 1 oz. (30 ml.) aloe vera gel
- 1 oz. (30 ml.) witch hazel extract
- 1 oz. (30 ml.) nettle extract
- 1/2 tsp. pantothenic acid (pro-Vitamin B5)
- 1/2 tsp. nicotinic acid (Vitamin B3)
- 1/2 tsp. ascorbic acid (Vitamin C)
- 1/2 tsp. Vitamin A palmitate
- 1/2 tsp. Vitamin E
- 1/2 tsp. modified lecithin
- 1 aspirin, dissolved in 1 tsp. hot water
- 30 drops rosemary PEO
- 30 drops lavender PEO

Mix all ingredients in a blender and place on high speed for one minute. Pour through a funnel into a glass bottle. To use, sprinkle drops onto the scalp, or saturate a cotton ball and blot over the scalp. Massage scalp gently but firmly until the tonic is absorbed (about 5 minutes). For best results, use daily.

AROMATIC ROSE VINEGAR

This French formula is used to relieve migraines as well as to clear the head and cleanse the scalp. Try it as a cold compress next time you feel feverish.

- full-blown roses, petals removed
- 1 oz. (30 ml.) apple cider vinegar
- 1 oz. (30 ml.) aloe vera gel
- 1 oz. (30 ml.) witch hazel extract
- 1 oz. (30 ml.) unflavored vodka
- distilled or spring water to cover petals
- 30 drops rose geranium PEO
- 10 drops rose absolute (optional)

Place the rose petals in a glass jar and pour the liquid ingredients (except the essential oil and absolute) over them to cover. Leave to steep for one week, then strain the liquid into a bowl, discarding the rose petals. Whisk the drops of essential oils and absolute into the liquid, and pour through a funnel into a bottle.

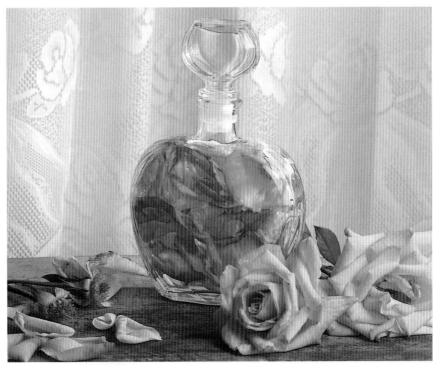

Hot Oil Treatments

One of the best things you can do for the health of your hair and scalp is to give yourself a natural hot oil treatment every week or two. Pick a convenient time, such as a weekend or a quiet evening when you can relax and allow the treatment time to work most effectively. A relaxing bath and nourishing face mask are two other options you can combine with your special scalp and hair treatment. Hot oil treatments work in several ways. First, the heat of the carrier oils loosens the scalp and hair follicles, allowing trapped sebum and old hairs to detach, freeing the scalp and follicles to benefit from special scalp massage. Second, through massage, the nutrients and active botanical elements in the aromatherapy oil are easily absorbed by the scalp follicles. Third, increased blood circulation to the scalp and stimulation of the follicles by massage and the oils result in accelerated healthy hair growth. Rubbing the oil through the scalp to the ends of the hair before shampooing also gives the hair a deep-conditioning treatment, leaving it full and vibrant, with a natural sheen and softness.

If your hair is naturally normal to oily, select cold-pressed oils such as sweet almond, grapeseed and hazelnut as a base, adding smaller amounts of heavier oils such as avocado, wheatgerm or jojoba. If your hair and scalp tend towards dryness, and you experience itchiness or flaking, increase the amounts of the latter three oils. Many people swear by jojoba oil, using it almost exclusively in their hot oil blends. Jojoba oil is molecularly comparable to human sebum, and is considered especially helpful for hair and scalp treatment. Avocado oil, a highly penetrative oil containing a wide range of beneficial vitamins and essential fatty acids, is an-

other oil that has specific hair- and scalp-regulating and nourishing abilities. Pure essential oils are a key additive to hot oil treatments. Lavender and rosemary oil are the classic oils to use for their cleansing, stimulating effects. If you have oily hair, try oils of cedarwood Atlas, lemon, juniper or pine in your blends. For a dry or sensitive scalp, sandalwood, neroli, sweet orange and ylang-ylang are excellent choices.

AROMATHERAPY HOT OIL TREATMENT

A lighter, penetrating oil mixture for weekly use if you have normal to oily hair.

- 2 oz. (60 ml.) sweet almond or hazelnut oil
- 1/2 oz. (15 ml.) avocado oil
- 1 tsp. (5 ml.) wheatgerm oil
- 1/2 tsp. modified lecithin
- 15 drops lavender PEO
- 15 drops rosemary PEO

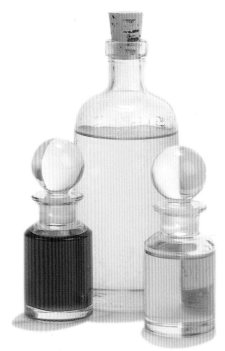

Mix the carrier oils and essential oils together in a small beaker, and pour into a glass bottle. Loosely cap the bottle and stand it in a mug half-full of just-boiled water to warm the oil. Part your hair in sections and apply oil to the scalp with a dropper or fingertips. Once your scalp is saturated, gently perform a firm, deep scalp massage using the pads of your fingertips in circular motions for 3 - 5 minutes. Wrap your hair in a towel and relax for 20 – 30 minutes. Shampoo your hair thoroughly, towel dry and style as usual.

ULTRA DEEP CONDITIONING HOT OIL TREATMENT

This richer formulation best suits those with dry, flaky or itchy scalp, and fine or brittle hair. Use every one to two weeks.

- 2 oz. (60 ml.) avocado oil
- 1 oz. (30 ml.) jojoba oil
- 1 tsp. (5 ml.) wheatgerm oil
- 1/2 tsp. modified lecithin
- 1/2 tsp. Vitamin E
- 1/2 tsp. Vitamin A
- 15 drops sandalwood PEO
- 15 drops sweet orange PEO
- 5 drops ylang-ylang PEO

Follow the directions given for the Aromatherapy Hot Oil Treatment.

Other carrier oils to try in custom hot oil treatments:
- macadamia nut
- kukui nut
- coconut
- peach kernel
- apricot kernel
- sesame
- sunflower
- safflower
- soybean

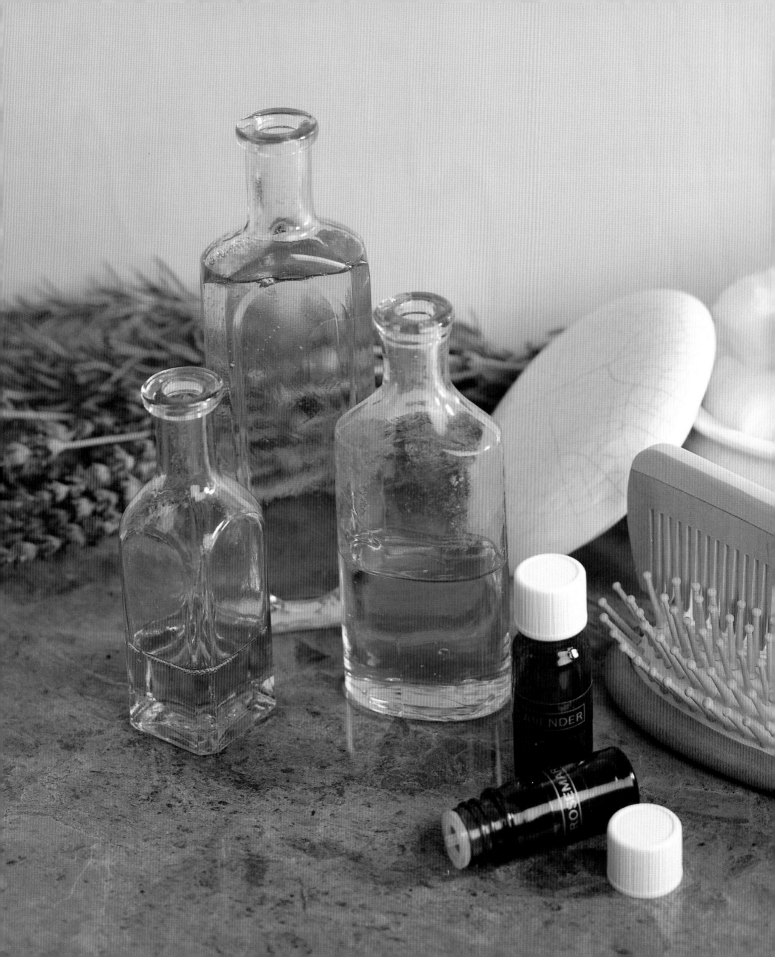

Chapter Five

Facial Skincare

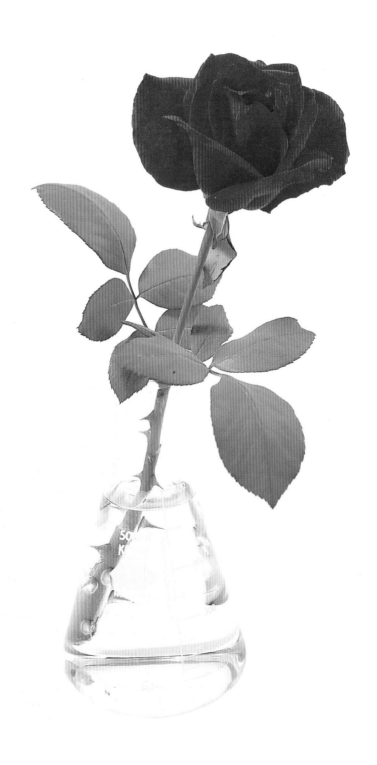

Introduction to Facial Skincare

Imagine creating your own all-natural facial cleansers, toners and moisturizers right at home, controlling the quality of the ingredients, adding healthful extracts and essences and customizing your creations to meet your skin's own unique needs. Making effective natural facial formulas yourself is simple once you have mastered a few basics, and the advantages are very real. You will be able to avoid synthetic chemicals, skin irritants and sensitizers present in many off-the-shelf cosmetic products. You will be choosing to spend your money, not on the packaging, advertising and promotion inherent in mass products, but on valuable, nutritious ingredients for the health and beauty of your skin. Your products will be cruelty-free and biodegradable, causing no harm to the environment or other living beings. Best of all, you will become familiar with a new world of healthy, natural ingredients, ranging from the simplest to the most sophisticated, learning how to use them to make dramatic improvements in the condition and appearance of your skin.

Pollution in our immediate environment and the continued proliferation of new chemicals into products we use everyday are causing inexplicable allergies and sensitivities in increasing numbers of people. Burning, reddening, dryness, severe itching, rashes and breakouts of the skin are the most common reactions to skin products. It is estimated that adverse reactions to commercial products account for 20,000 emergency room visits a year in the USA. Given the high permeability of the skin, there is also the concern of unseen damage done by potent systemic toxins. The FDA has long been concerned with the issue of contaminants and toxins that are created in synthetic materials used in the cosmetic manufacturing process. Certain categories of standard ingredients in synthesis can create nitrosamines, dangerous substances that have proven to cause cancer in laboratory animals. Dermatological specialists acknowledge that a large percentage of ingredients in commercial skincare products pose some degree of health risk. Harsh surfactants (liquid soap bases), chemical solubilizers and emulsifiers, and synthetic fragrances are the main culprits. Sensitivities to these ingredients are common in the general population. Natural ingredients, on the other hand, have been safely and effectively used for thousands of years, and a wealth of information exists on their use in skincare. Once you are familiar with the cosmetic and therapeutic qualities of natural materials, you will trust them to safely and holistically balance and nourish your skin.

With so many commercial cosmetic products available and the accompanying persuasive advertising, it is often easy to believe that this year's 'miracle ingredient' will work wonders. Too often, disillusion soon sets in when the product fails to deliver, or, to add insult to injury, causes problems worse than those it was purchased to solve! Take control of this situation by learning to understand the ingredients in cosmetics as described in the product labeling. Several excellent books are available to help you research those unpronounceable technical names (consult your local book store). Often these ingredients are not nearly as intimidating as they appear. For those with allergies and skin sensitivities, self-education is a necessity, and with a little detective work, the offending substances can be discovered and avoided. Your best choices then are to find a natural product line especially developed for holistic skincare, or to learn to make your own all-natural, customized skincare products yourself at home.

When making natural cosmetics, you will be using nutritious food-grade materials – cold-pressed vegetable, nut and seed oils, distilled or spring water, floral waters, fruits, bio-active herbal extracts and pure essential oils, vitamins and precious oils and essences. Many treatments, like facial steaming, exfoliating and clarifying, combine fresh ingredients which are activated once prepared. When customizing your formulas, you can choose to use them fresh (meaning that your products will require refrigeration) or to add a small amount of preservative to give them an extended shelf life (see 'A Word About Preservation' on page 15). Cleansers and moisturizers, being oil and water emulsions, require preservation to prevent long-term spoilage. Water-based products can be preserved through the addition of alcohol, tincture of benzoin, water-soluble vitamins or grapefruit seed extract. Oil-based products need anti-oxidant Vitamin E and essential oils to extend their shelf life. In the following recipes, you will learn which ingredients are valuable for your skin type in each category. So, whether your skin is oily or blemished or dry and sensitive, you can customize an individual formula to meet your own skincare needs. In addition to the sense of satisfaction you will feel from making your own custom facial skincare products yourself, you will also have created something of lasting value – the awareness of how to take control of the health, beauty and well-being of your skin!

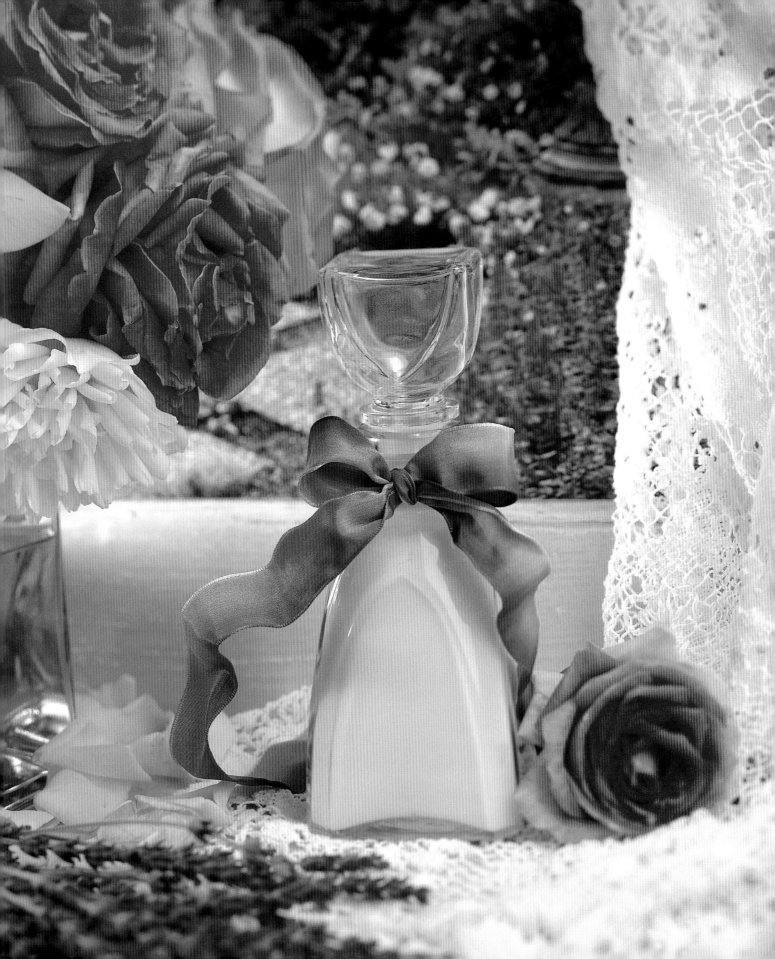

Cleansing Milks and Lotions

The first step in your natural beauty program is to thoroughly cleanse your delicate facial skin without stripping it of its natural oils or disturbing its protective acid mantle. Pure water is the best skin cleanser, but it does not remove surface dirt, excess oil, makeup residue, dead skin cells or environmental pollutants — for this a cleansing additive is necessary. Preferences for soap-based cleansers or emulsion-type cleansers are personal and are based on skin type and past experience with cleansing products. Generally, soaps or foaming cleansers are most effective for those with young, oily or blemished skin. For other skin types, surfactants in many commercial soaps temporarily disturb the hydrolipid layer of the skin and can lead to increased sensitivity, dryness and susceptibility to dermatological problems. For all skin types other than oily, gentle cleansing milks — light combinations of water, natural emollients, emulsifiers and preservatives, and special botanical ingredients — are the best choice. Pure essential oils can be added for their fragrance and cleansing, healing properties.

To maximize the effectiveness of your cleansing routine, thoroughly wash your face and neck first with warm water to relax muscles, soften skin and loosen dirt particles and old skin cells. If wearing makeup, carefully remove it with cotton balls saturated with lotion. Using a clean washcloth every day will help hydrate your skin and prepare it for cleansing. Work the cleanser gently over the skin with your fingertips or cotton balls for one minute. Rinse thoroughly with warm water until all cleanser is removed and your skin feels moist and smooth. Splash with cool water and pat your skin lightly dry with a clean towel.

GENTLE FOAMING CLEANSER

For those who prefer a soap-based cleanser, here is a mild yet effective formula for everyday use.

- *4 oz. (120 ml.) unfragranced liquid coconut soap*
- *1 oz. (30 ml.) liquid unpasteurized honey*
- *1 oz. (30 ml.) aloe vera gel*
- *1 oz. (30 ml.) sweet almond oil*

Add essential oils as follows:
For normal to oily skin, add:

- *80 drops ylang-ylang PEO*

For oily, problem skin, substitute:

- *40 drops lemon PEO*
- *40 drops rosemary PEO*

Mix all ingredients together in a glass measuring cup, stir well, and pour into a bottle with pump dispenser. Shake before each use. Work up a lather and then rinse thoroughly with warm water.

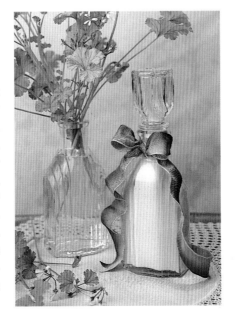

LAVENDER AND ROSE CLEANSING MILK

A fragrant and soothing milky emulsion with aromatherapeutic benefits. Lavender essential oil and rose absolute are specific for normal, dry, mature or dehydrated skin. The soft, delicate aroma of fresh flowers lingers after cleansing.

- *8 oz. (240 ml.) basic unfragranced cleansing milk (see Chapter Three)*
- *30 drops lavender PEO*
- *10 drops rose absolute*

Pour the unfragranced lotion into a small glass mixing bowl or beaker. Add the essential oil and absolute slowly, stirring continuously. When the ingredients are fully blended, pour into a glass bottle. Apply as needed.

ROSE GERANIUM CLEANSING MILK WITH YLANG-YLANG AND CEDARWOOD

A light yet penetrating lotion for removing excess oil and regulating skin metabolism. Geranium, ylang-ylang and cedarwood are excellent essential oils for balancing oily, unpredictable and over-active skin, and they impart a fresh, floral aroma to the cleansing milk.

- *8 oz. (240 ml.) basic unfragranced cleansing milk (see Chapter Three)*
- *30 drops rose geranium PEO*
- *20 drops cedarwood Atlas PEO*
- *10 drops ylang-ylang PEO*

Pour the unfragranced lotion into a small glass mixing bowl or beaker. Add the essential oils drop by drop, stirring continuously. When the ingredients are fully blended, pour into a glass bottle. Apply as needed.

Facial Toners and Astringents

After cleansing face and neck, applying a refreshing liquid toner is the second step towards healthy, balanced skin. As is the case with facial cleansers, toners can be customized to satisfy individual skin needs. Natural toners are aqueous (water-based) solutions that have the ability to be quite astringent (through the addition of a distilled alcohol such as vodka and certain herbal distillates) or very mild and healing (through the inclusion of floral waters, hydrosols and herbal infusions.) The primary purpose of a facial toner is to remove all final traces of cleanser, excess sebum and makeup residue, while reducing pore size and restoring a neutral pH balance to the skin. An effective toner also prepares the skin to absorb active principles — beneficial herbal extracts, pure essential oils, essential fatty acids, vitamins and other nutrients. The ideal toner supports the continuous efforts of delicate facial skin to resist environmental and other stressors, repair itself and regenerate healthy new   skin cells.

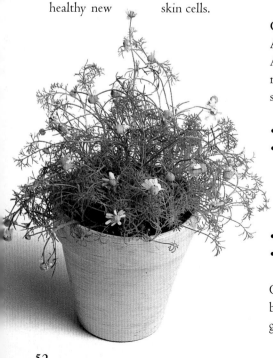

Every great beauty of times past attributed her unique charms to her own secret 'cosmetic water' formula. These recipes were basically toners concocted of fruits, flowers or herbs in a fresh solution of water, vinegar or alcohol. Most renowned is the famous 'Hungary Water,' a rosemary and citrus wine infusion created in the fourteenth century by Isabella, Queen of Hungary, a septuagenarian whose beauty ignited a 'burning passion' in a neighboring 18-year old prince who subsequently proposed marriage to her! Many stories exist of the powers of similar beauties throughout the centuries, proving the abilities of natural ingredients to enhance health and beauty in eras lacking refrigeration, preservation, 'miracle ingredients' or other scientific discoveries. Facial toners require little or no preservation and are extremely easy to make. With a little practice, you can customize toners to your own skin type, choosing from a wide range of natural and inexpensive plant-based ingredients.

GENTLE CHAMOMILE AND ALOE VERA TONER

A mild, cooling gel-like formula which removes redness and soothes inflamed skin. For dry, sensitive skin.

- *4 oz. (120 ml.) distilled or spring water*
- *2 oz. (60 ml.) aloe vera gel*
- *2 oz. (60 ml.) infused chamomile tea*
- *1 tsp. xanthan gum powder*
- *1/2 tsp. grapefruit seed extract*
- *1/4 tsp. evening primrose oil*
- *8 drops Roman chamomile PEO*
- *2 drops rose absolute (optional)*

Combine all ingredients in a blender, blend briefly on low setting, pour into a glass bottle, and cap. Use as needed.

SPARKLING CITRUS FACIAL TONER

This refreshing toner includes Vitamin C and citrus oils to cleanse and enliven dull skin. For normal to oily skin.

- *4 oz. (120 ml.) sparkling mineral water*
- *2 oz. (60 ml.) aloe vera gel*
- *2 oz. (60 ml.) witch hazel extract*
- *1/2 tsp. polysorbate 20*
- *1/4 tsp. Vitamin C powder*
- *20 drops grapefruit PEO*
- *10 drops lemon PEO*
- *10 drops sweet orange PEO*

Combine all ingredients in a glass measuring cup, stir well, pour into a glass bottle, and cap. For best results, shake well before each use.

HERBAL BALANCING ASTRINGENT

A therapeutic toner containing active ingredients to detoxify, control outbreaks and encourage healthy skin cell turnover. For oily or problem skin.

- *4 oz. (120 ml.) distilled or spring water*
- *2 oz. (60 ml.) aloe vera gel*
- *1 oz. (30 ml.) unfiltered apple cider vinegar*
- *1 oz. (30 ml.) 90-proof unflavored vodka*
- *1/2 tsp. polysorbate 20*
- *1/2 tsp. grapefruit seed extract*
- *10 drops tea tree PEO*
- *10 drops juniper berry PEO*
- *10 drops rosemary PEO*
- *10 drops lavender PEO*

Combine all ingredients in a glass measuring cup, and stir well with a wire whisk until the ingredients are fully blended. Pour into a glass bottle, and cap. Shake well before each use.

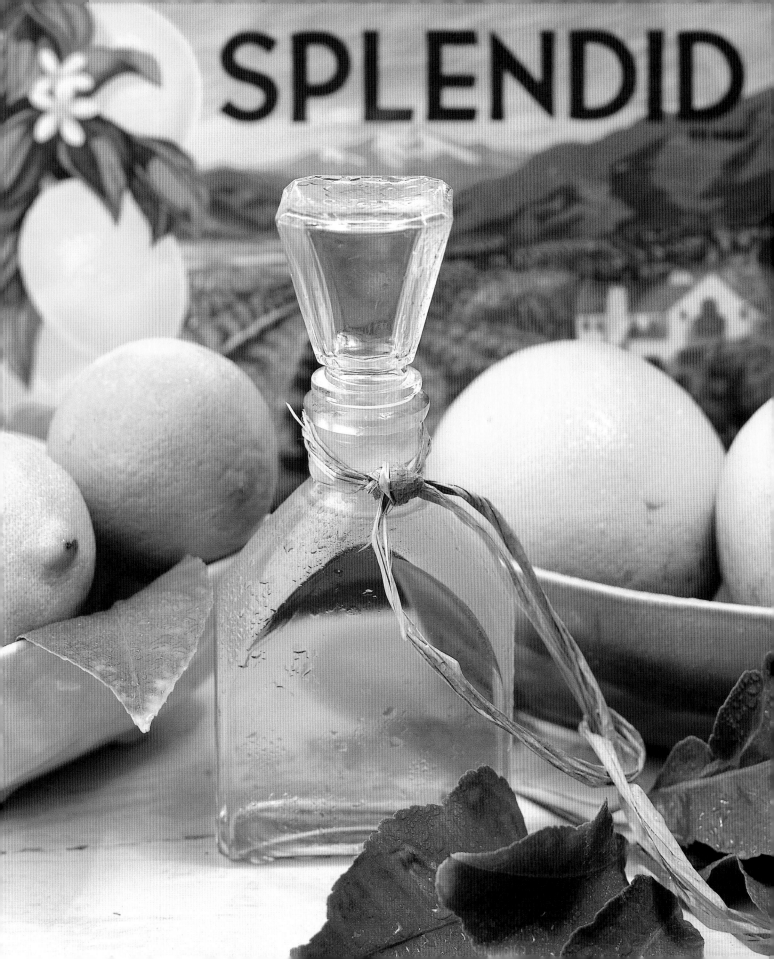

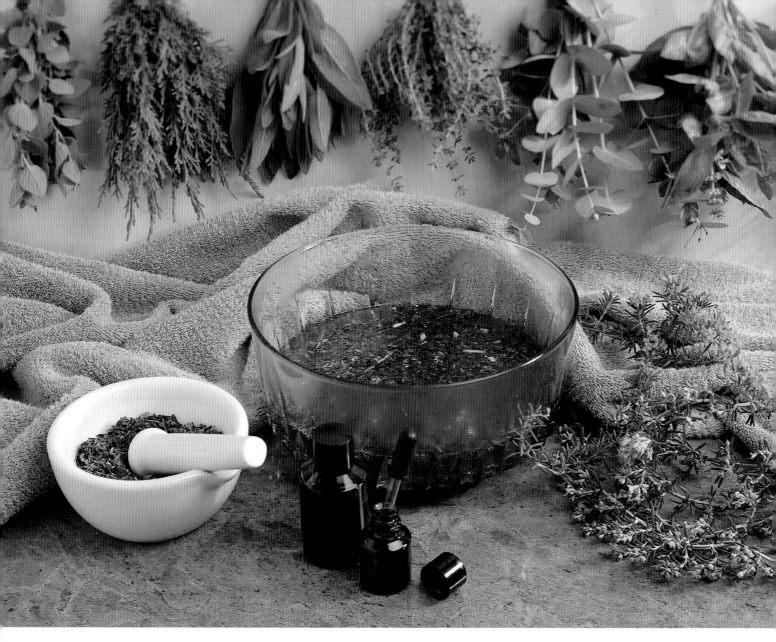

HERBS AND ESSENTIAL OILS FOR FACIAL STEAMING, BY SKIN TYPE

For dry, sensitive skin:

- lavender
- chamomile
- rose geranium
- melissa
- rose
- jasmine
- orange blossom
- elder flower
- parsley
- meadowsweet
- patchouli

For normal skin:

- lavender
- rosemary
- rose geranium
- melissa
- chamomile
- rose
- peppermint
- marigold
- sweet orange
- sandalwood
- comfrey

For oily, over-active skin:

- rosemary
- eucalyptus
- sweet basil
- peppermint
- marjoram
- thyme
- lemon verbena
- cedarwood
- lemongrass
- petitgrain
- sage

For blemished, acneic skin:

- eucalyptus
- thyme
- tea tree
- juniper
- cypress
- yarrow
- pine
- fir
- lemon
- niaouli
- cajeput

Facial Steaming Herbs

Facial steaming (also known as 'facial sauna') is one of the oldest, simplest ways to thoroughly deep-cleanse your skin. The moist, warm vapor produced by the steam relaxes tense muscles, stimulates glandular and lymphatic activity, loosens congestion in the head, clears sinuses, increases circulation, oxygenates and hydrates the skin and stimulates skin cell regeneration. In addition to clearing the skin of any remaining dirt, oil, makeup and loosened skin cells, a good facial steam encourages sweating so that deep-seated toxins and impurities are released through the pores. Through the centuries, people have added herbs indigenous to the area to the steaming water to experience their individual qualities. Now, we can also choose from a wide array of pure essential oils which can be added by the drop to the steaming water, with or without herbs. In addition to their physical actions, pure essential oils have psycho-aromatherapeutic benefits which can be felt when they are added to the steaming water and directly inhaled. The small amounts of essential oils needed for this make facial steaming one of the most economical and effective ways to enjoy true aromatherapy!

To create the ultimate aromatherapy facial steam treatment, place a large handful of your chosen herbs into a large glass or ceramic bowl and pour two quarts of boiling water over them. Wait a few moments for the initial steam to subside, gently stir the herbs, and then add 2 - 6 drops total of pure essential oils. Sit comfortably with your face over the bowl and drape a large towel like a tent over your head and the steambath. If the steam is too intense, lift the towel slightly to allow it to escape. Keep your face at a comfortable distance for the duration of the treatment, breathing slowly and deeply. After the treatment, rinse your face and neck thoroughly with warm water and gently rub a clean, damp washcloth in circular motions over your face to complete the cleansing process. Allow your skin time to return to its normal temperature, pat dry with a clean towel and apply a light moisturizer.

DEEP CLEANSING HERBAL STEAM WITH PURIFYING OILS

Customize your own facial steam treatment using herbs and/or essential oils specific to your own skin type. The herbs and the pure essential oils derived from them (listed opposite) are detoxifying and antibacterial, and have a deep-cleansing, toning and firming effect on the skin, while promoting the growth of healthy new skin cells.

- *One large handful mixed dried herbs*
- *6 drops total PEOs or blend*

Follow the directions for giving yourself an aromatherapeutic facial steam.

ELIZABETHAN FLORAL FACIAL STEAM

A delicately fragrant mixture of flowers and herbs used since Elizabethan times to cleanse, soften and hydrate facial skin. For dry, sensitive or mature skin.

- *One handful equal parts of lavender, rose, chamomile, melissa, elder flower, calendula and lemon verbena*
- *1-2 drops of either lavender, melissa or chamomile PEO, or rose absolute*

Follow the directions for giving yourself an aromatherapeutic facial steam. For dry skin, facial steaming once or twice a month is recommended.

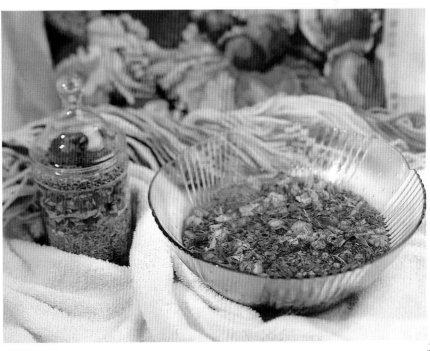

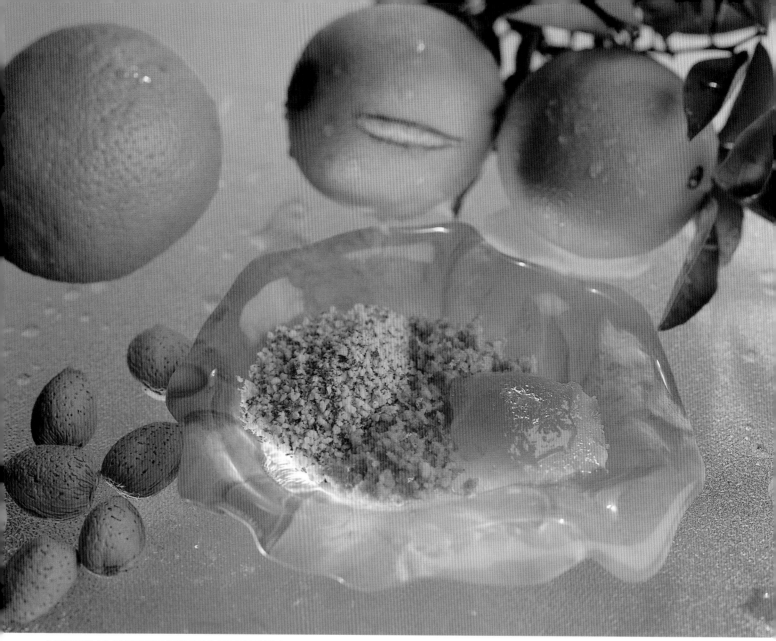

NATURAL EXFOLIATING MATERIALS

For normal to dry skin:

- ground oatmeal
- oat bran
- ground almonds
- cornmeal
- wheatgerm
- powdered milk
- rice bran
- strawberries
- grain flours
- ground herbs and
  herbal powders

For oily or problem skin:

- ground orange peel
- ground lemon peel
- sugar
- oatmeal
- lecithin granules
- fine-ground coffee
- psyllium husks
- small-textured cereal
  grains, e.g., amaranth
- fibrous fruit,
  e.g., pineapple

NATURAL CARRIER MATERIALS

For normal to dry skin:

- distilled/spring water
- mineral water
- milk
- cream
- honey
- vegetable glycerin
- floral hydrosols
- rose water
- cooled herbal teas
- cold-pressed oils

For oily or problem skin:

- yogurt
- buttermilk
- kefir
- apple cider vinegar
- witch hazel
- vodka
- honey
- orange flower water
- herbal vinegar
- aloe vera gel
- cooled herbal infusions

Scrubs and Exfoliants

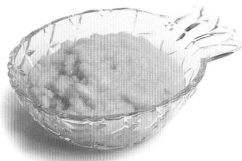

The old-fashioned term 'scrub' has been largely replaced with new concepts in cosmetic science, such as bio-active peeling substances, specialized masks, vegetal extracts, glycolic and alpha-hydroxy acids, and a host of other exotic products and methods promising spectacular results. The basic concept behind all these treatments is the same — the mechanical removal of dead or damaged skin cells from the uppermost layer of the skin. Facial skin is composed of three layers; the subcutaneous layer, the dermis and the epidermis. The epidermis, or protective outer layer, is divided into the basal (germinating) layer, where new young skin cells are constantly being created, and the protective horny (external) layer. The young cells move continuously upward through the epidermis, eventually becoming part of the horny layer. At the last stages of the growth cycle, the uppermost cells become scaly and detach themselves. Our facial skin is being endlessly renewed in this cycle, which takes approximately 28 days. Scrubs, exfoliants and the newer cosmetic treatments provide a physical means to assist the skin in sloughing off dead skin cells, clarifying the complexion and stimulating new cell growth. Care should always be taken, though, to ensure that the exfoliation process is not as extreme as to damage the skin during its natural cycle of regeneration.

To exfoliate, cleanse skin thoroughly with warm water and pat dry. Mix 1 Tbsp. of your selected natural exfoliating material in a small bowl with 1 Tbsp. of natural carrier. Add a little unpasteurized honey to the mixture to achieve a smooth, creamy consistency. Apply the mixture to the skin with fingertips, working over the nose, chin, jawline, cheekbones and forehead with small, firm circular motions. After massaging for several minutes, rinse off all traces of exfoliating material with warm water, pat skin dry and moisturize lightly.

CLASSIC ORANGE/ALMOND/HONEY SCRUB

A fresh, home-made alternative to commercial scrub products. The orange peel contains citric acid and Vitamin C, and the ground almond meal and honey are excellent for softening the skin. For all skin types.

- *1 Tbsp. fresh grated orange peel*
- *1 Tbsp. ground almond meal*
- *1 Tbsp. unpasteurized honey*
- *10 drops sweet orange PEO*
- *distilled water (as needed)*

Mix the ingredients together in a small bowl and apply to damp face and neck. Use small circular motions and then rinse thoroughly. Pat dry and follow with a light moisturizer. In addition to exfoliation with scrubs, an excellent skin regenerator is papaya, which contains papain, a potent enzyme which 'digests' dead skin cells while leaving live ones untouched. Bromelain, the enzyme in pineapple, performs a similar function. By combining these two powerful fruit enzymes, you can make a bio-active peeling mask at home!

PAPAYA AND PINEAPPLE EXFOLIATING TREATMENT

A natural fruit mixture with vitamin C to remove dead skin cells, lighten age spots and reveal younger skin with a healthy glow. For all skin types.

- *2 Tbsp. mashed papaya*
- *2 Tbsp. mashed fresh pineapple*
- *1 Tbsp. unpasteurized honey*
- *1/2 tsp. Vitamin C powder*
- *6 drops sweet orange PEO*

Select under-ripe papaya and over-ripe pineapple for the highest enzyme activity. Combine the mashed fruits and other ingredients in a small bowl. Work mixture gently over the skin for one minute, then apply a layer and leave for 3-5 minutes. Rinse thoroughly and splash with cool water.

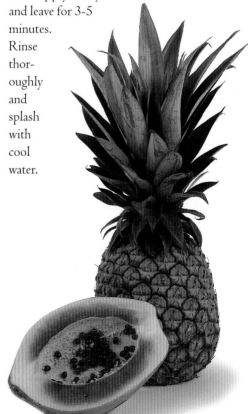

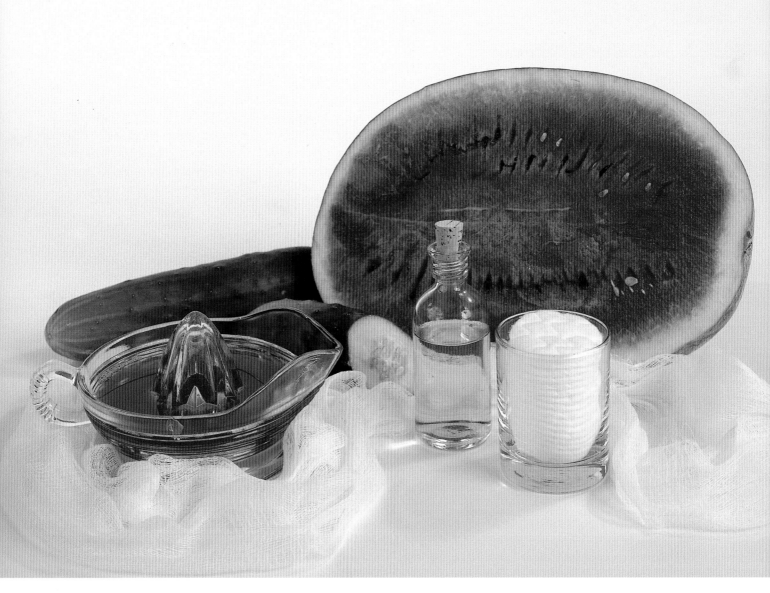

FRESH JUICES FOR FACIAL TREATMENTS, BY SKIN TYPE

For dry, dehydrated skin:

- canteloupe
- honeydew melon
- peach
- nectarine
- pear
- papaya
- apple
- watermelon
- black cherry
- mango

For normal skin:

- apple
- cucumber
- watermelon
- strawberry
- papaya
- sweet citrus, e.g. mandarin
- carrot
- pineapple
- grape

For oily or problem skin:

- bitter greens, e.g., dandelion, watercress
- cabbage
- acidic citrus, e.g. grapefruit, lemon
- cranberry
- pineapple
- tomato
- celery
- spinach

For troubled, acneic skin:

- acidic citrus, e.g., lemon, lime
- bitter greens, e.g., dandelion, watercress
- super greens, e.g., wheatgrass, barley shoots
- radish
- ginger
- onion
- garlic

Clarifying Treatments

In recent years, cosmetic scientists have discovered that important skin-clarifying factors, known as alpha-hydroxy and beta-hydroxy acids, are available in abundance in everyday fruits and vegetables. Glycolic acid is derived from sugar cane; citric acid, from citrus fruits and red berries; malic acid, from apples, apricots and other fruits; and lactic acid, from tomatoes and other sources. These biological substances are of great interest in skincare, as in low concentrations, they moisturize the skin and make it pliable, while in higher concentrations, they provide an exfoliating and peeling effect, clarifying and smoothing the complexion.

Additionally, most fruits and vegetables are excellent sources of vitamins, minerals, amino acids, enzymes and chlorophyll. Enzymes are important in desquamation (peeling) of dead skin cells, while chlorophyll is a potent cleanser, tonic and cell stimulator. Carrot and green juices are high in beta-carotene (pro-Vitamin A) while sprout juices contain high amounts of Vitamin B complex. All fresh juices are excellent sources of Vitamin C, and celery, beet and green juices contain anti-oxidant Vitamin E. Recent studies have shown that the epidermis is able to absorb vitamins and nutrients from topically applied liquid juice solutions, greatly benefiting the strength, elasticity and general appearance of the skin. Facial formulas of olden days instinctively utilized this knowledge, and fresh fruits and vegetables were often included in recipes. For best results, if you are truly seeking improvements in your skin's condition, purchase a juicer and make juices from the list opposite, drinking them

often as well as using them in face washes. While expensive skin products containing alpha-hydroxy acids have flooded the commercial market, with a little time, ingenuity and an electric juicer, you can make this effective, pure alpha hydroxy acid plant juice at home from all-natural sources to use in your facial treatments.

ALPHA HYDROXY ACID CLARIFYING FACIAL LIQUID

Use this juice directly to exfoliate the skin, or mix with water to make a mild clarifying toner.

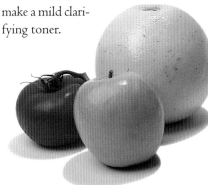

- *1 large ripe grapefruit, peeled*
- *1 large green apple, peeled and cored*
- *1 large ripe red tomato*
- *1/2 tsp. grapefruit seed extract*

Wash the fruits and chop them into large pieces. Pass all the pieces through an electric juicer, collecting the mixed juices in a measuring cup. Filter the juice through a coffee filter, and add the grapefruit seed extract. Pour into a glass bottle and refrigerate for use as needed. To use, saturate cotton balls and apply over face and neck, avoiding eye area and lips. After five minutes, splash the skin clean with warm water.

Juicy fruits have a high purified liquid content and bioenergetic factors which make them perfect for washing the skin.

Many different skin problems can benefit from a regular fruit juice 'wash.' Refer to the chart opposite to select juices appropriate to your skin type. Use an electric juicer to make the freshest juices for greatest effectiveness.

WATERMELON AND CUCUMBER CLARIFYING TONER

A wonderfully refreshing, cooling liquid for all skin types. The two juices combined with the slightly astringent witch hazel extract and the hint of peppermint have a cleansing, energizing effect on the skin.

- *1 small cucumber, cut in 1" sections*
- *1 segment ripe watermelon*
- *2 Tbsp. witch hazel extract*
- *2 Tbsp. mineral water*
- *1 drop peppermint PEO*

Squeeze the juice from the ripe fruits using a lemon squeezer. Strain through a sieve or cheesecloth into a small bowl. Add the witch hazel and stir. Use cotton pads to dampen the face and neck, saturating the skin with the solution. For an intensive clarifying treatment, cut a piece of cheesecloth the size of your face, with openings for nose and mouth. Saturate the cheesecloth with the liquid and lay it over your face for five minutes. Finish by splashing the skin clean with warm water and drying gently with a clean towel. During the hot summer months, this mixture will keep your skin refreshed and hydrated, particularly if you add a couple of ice cubes to the toner before applying to your skin. This mixture is best used fresh, but if you want to keep it for a short time in the refrigerator, add one tablespoon of unflavored vodka to each four ounces of juice.

Masks and Corrective Treatments

Clays from the earth are the oldest skin cleansers known to man. Their fine texture, absorbency and high mineral content make them indispensable for deep-cleaning the skin, drawing out toxins and impurities, removing oil, dead skin cells and surface dirt, and balancing and correcting over-active skin conditions. There are many types of facial clays to choose from — the soft green French clay, white kaolin clay from China, rose pink Moroccan clay, off-white bentonite, pale gray fuller's earth, or olive-green, mineral-rich sea clay. The special qualities of purified clays are activated once liquids have been added to make a thick, creamy paste. Clays are also an excellent medium for the addition of healing herbal powders, pure essential oils and vitamins. The active botanical elements and nutrients are absorbed by the skin while the mask is drying, resulting in an intensive balancing and rejuvenating treatment for the skin.

To make a personalized facial mask, mix equal parts of the clay of your choice with the liquids of your choice (see 'Natural Carrier Materials' in the Scrubs and Exfoliants section,) adding several drops of pure essential oils for their fragrance and aromatherapeutic benefits.

ACTIVE BOTANICAL MASK WITH PURIFYING OILS

This mask is designed for the skin type most in need of deep-cleansing and balancing —over-active, oily, acneic or blemished skin.

- *1 Tbsp. green clay powder*
- *1 tsp. plain yogurt*
- *1 tsp. unpasteurized honey*
- *1/4 tsp. St. John's Wort powder*
- *1/4 tsp. goldenseal powder*
- *2 drops clary sage PEO*
- *2 drops white thyme PEO*
- *2 drops lavender PEO*

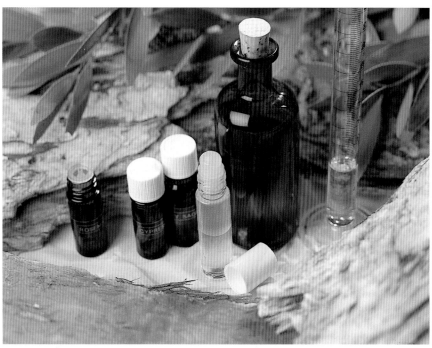

Mix all ingredients together slowly in a small bowl or cup to form a smooth paste. Add more liquid if the paste is too dry; more clay if the mixture is too liquid. Apply gently to the skin with clean fingertips and leave on for 10 - 15 minutes. Rinse off thoroughly with water and pat dry with a clean towel.

CORRECTIVE TREATMENTS

Oily, problem skins prone to breakout often need immediate attention to prevent the spread of infection and further breakouts. The antibacterial, antifungal and antiviral properties of certain essential oils make them the perfect choice for controlling blemishes and stimulating healthy skin cell growth. Herbal tinctures in an alcohol base have excellent drying, disinfecting and healing qualities. Together, they create a remarkable solution for dramatically clearing up blemished skin in a very short time.

MELALEUCA BLEMISH PEN

This watery liquid contains three potent essential oils from the Melaleuca tree family with other oils in the base of astringent yarrow herb.

- *1 tsp. (5 ml.) tincture of yarrow*
- *20 drops tea tree PEO*
- *20 drops cajeput PEO*
- *20 drops niaouli PEO*
- *20 drops clary sage PEO*
- *20 drops rosemary PEO*

Mix all ingredients together in a 1/3 oz. (10 ml.) bottle or roller ball pen type applicator vial, and shake well. As the liquids will naturally separate, shake well to activate before each use. Apply a small dab directly to the blemish.

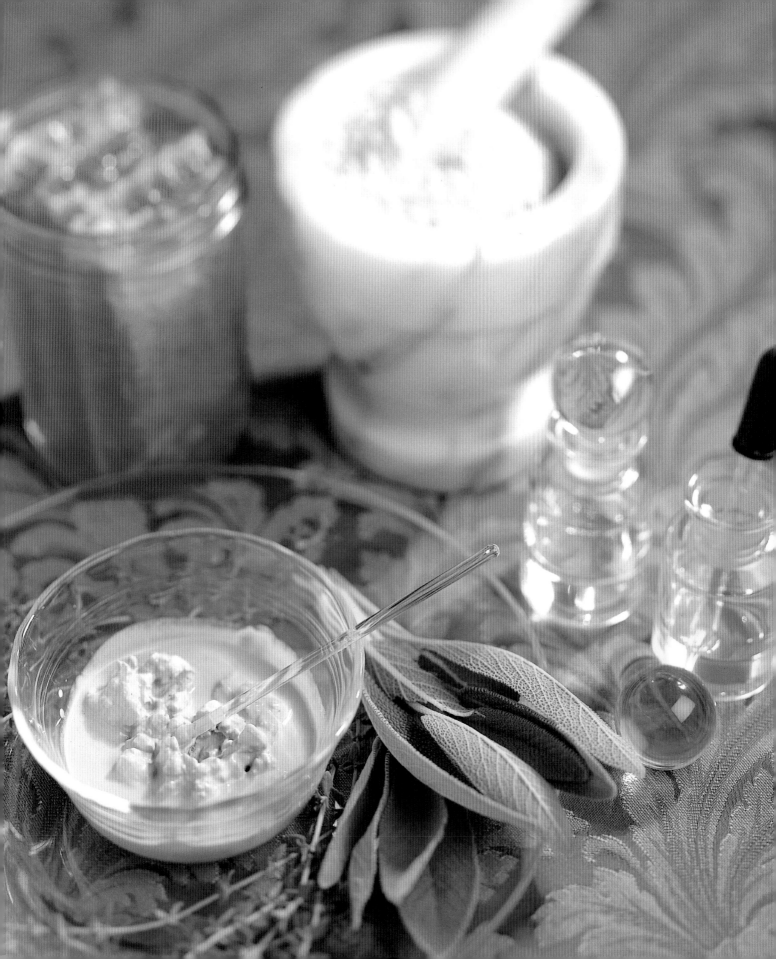

Special Eye Treatments

The delicate area around the eyes deserves special care — having few oil or sweat glands, skin around the eyes is the first to show aging, and is very sensitive to incorrect handling or neglect. Eye muscles are constantly moving, even during sleep, and facial expressions like squinting and frowning stress the thin, sensitive skin, as do lack of sleep, poor diet, hormonal changes, allergies, and too-vigorous makeup application and removal. Despite its relative inability to retain moisture, the delicate skin of the eye also cannot tolerate over-rich creams and will react quickly with puffiness, whiteheads, sensitivity and irritation.

Simple, old-fashioned remedies are surprisingly effective. A key ingredient in many natural eye care treatments is Roman chamomile (Chamaemelum nobile,) familiar to everyone for its cheerful daisy-like flowers and fruity-herbal aroma, like ripe apples. For centuries, chamomile flowers, both fresh and dried, have been infused as a tea to wash the skin and soothe tired, inflamed eyes. Chamomile is particularly rich in the potent anti-inflammatory substances azulene, chamazulene and bisabolol.

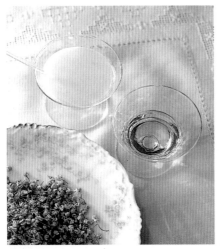

Treat your 'windows of the soul' to a little care and attention. Stress, travel, harsh lighting and glare, and long hours at the computer or on the road exact their toll in the form of 'bags,' dark circles, bleary red eyes and a dull, tired appearance. Basic eye compresses made from cooled chamomile tea bags are excellent for reducing puffiness and brightening the eyes.

THE SIMPLEST PICK-ME-UP EYE TREATMENT

- *2 chamomile tea bags*
- *8 oz. (240 ml.) spring water*

Bring the water to a boil, pour over the tea bags in a large cup, steep for one minute, remove tea bags, and place them in the freezer for five minutes while you sip the tea. Place the cool tea bags over your eyes, lie back and relax. This quick, simple treatment is guaranteed to totally de-stress you and bring a lively sparkle to your eyes!

GENTLE CHAMOMILE EYE MAKEUP REMOVER

A soft, light, creamy liquid which thoroughly removes makeup while gently moisturizing the skin.

- *1 oz. (30 ml.) basic moisturizing cream (see Chapter Three)*
- *1 oz. (30 ml.) cooled chamomile tea*
- *1 oz. (30 ml.) sweet almond oil*
- *1 oz. (30 ml.) aloe vera gel*
- *1/4 tsp. grapefruit seed extract*
- *6 drops Roman chamomile PEO*

Mix all ingredients in a small bowl and stir thoroughly with a small whisk until fully blended, Pour into a glass bottle. Keep in a cool place; apply as needed.

Another valuable botanical for eye care is green tea (Camellia sinensis.) Prepared in the same manner as chamomile tea, green tea contains tannins, polyphenols and anti-oxidants to tone and tighten the skin. Aloe vera gel has a soothing and firming effect on delicate skin.

GREEN TEA AND CHAMOMILE EYE GEL

A soothing and restorative gel for face, neck and eyes. For all skin types.

- *4 oz. (120 ml.) aloe vera gel*
- *2 oz. (60 ml.) chamomile tea, cooled*
- *2 oz. (60 ml.) green tea, cooled*
- *1 tsp. xanthan gum powder*
- *1 tsp. grapefruit seed extract*
- *12 drops Roman chamomile PEO*

As the chamomile tea and green tea are cooling, stir in the xanthan gum powder. Add the aloe vera gel and chamomile essential oil, and stir the mixture occasionally until cool. Refrigerate briefly if desired. Apply the gel whenever you are feeling eye strain or tiredness. After 5 - 10 minutes, rinse off with cool water.

ELEGANT CHAMOMILE EYE CREAM

A fine-textured cream formulated especially for care of the skin around the eyes. For all skin types.

- *2 oz. (60 ml.) basic moisturizing cream (see Chapter Three)*
- *4 drops Roman chamomile PEO*
- *2 drops jasmine absolute (optional)*

Mix all ingredients together in a small bowl. Spoon into a sterile glass jar, seal and keep in a cool place. Massage a little around the eyes as needed.

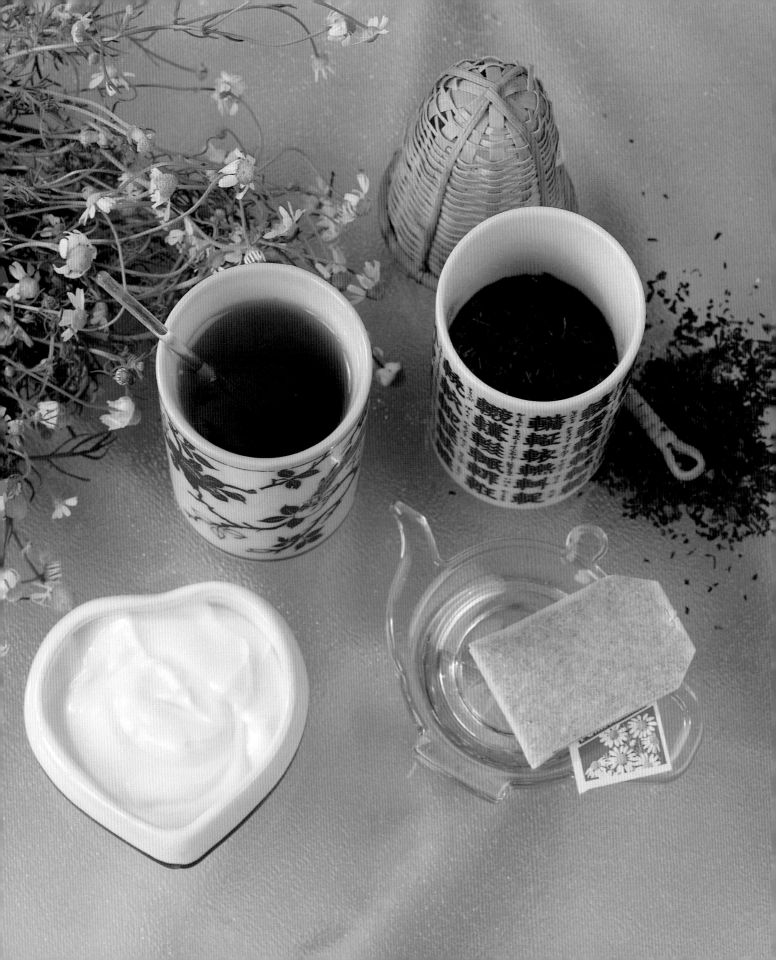

Moisturizing Creams

After cleansing and toning, the most important step in natural skincare is moisturizing — nourishing your skin and replacing lost moisture, oils and nutrients. Centuries ago, skin creams were made by combining oil, wax, water and alkaline salts. 'Cold cream' was thought to have originated in the second century AD, when the renowned Greek physician Galen recorded a formula containing olive oil and beeswax. Updated versions of this recipe use lighter cold-pressed oils, floral waters, vitamins and essential oils to produce a rich moisture cream for everyday use. The advantage of this basic cream is that it contains none of the occlusive or potentially allergenic ingredients often found in commercial products, and it can be customized with special bio-active ingredients to suit the needs of your skin type.

A nourishing natural moisturizing cream is an emulsion composed of distilled or spring water, cold-pressed vegetable, nut or seed oils, specialty oils or butters, vitamins and essential oils, with a preservative to ensure freshness. Moisturizing creams can also contain liposomes to add to their effectiveness. Liposomes can be generated in home-made creams by using special ingredients including phospholipids (from lecithin) and mixing the creams at high speeds in a small electric blender. A liposome cream formula is given in Chapter Three. Make your creams up in small batches; set aside one to two ounces for immediate use, and refrigerate the rest. Your home-made cream will be rich and nutritious, free of unnecessary chemicals, synthetic fragrance or additives. Within a few weeks of use, you'll be truly amazed at the difference in your skin's appearance and texture!

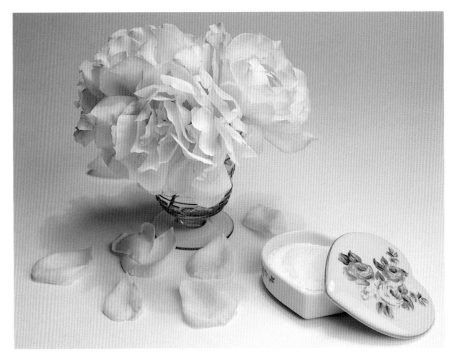

CLASSIC DEEP MOISTURIZING CREAM OF ROSES

Galen's original formula has been modernized to include rose water and essential oils. Excellent for all skin types.

- *1 Tbsp. beeswax*
- *4 oz. (120 ml.) cold-pressed oil*
- *2 oz. (60 ml.) distilled water*
- *2 tsp. (10 ml.) rose water*
- *1/4 tsp. borax powder*
- *20 drops rose geranium oil*
- *6 drops rose absolute (optional)*

Combine the beeswax and carrier oil in a bain-marie and heat gently until liquid. Stir the borax into the water and bring to a boil. Immediately whisk the water into the oil until blended. The mixture will acquire a creamy consistency and thicken as it cools. Add the rose water, essential oils and rose absolute, and stir well. Spoon the cream into several small clean jars.

NOURISHING MOISTURE CREAM

This velvety, skin-smoothing formula is enriched with added vitamins and precious essences. A real delight for dry, dehydrated or mature skin types.

- *1 oz. (30 ml.) basic moisturizing cream (see Chapter Three)*
- *1/4 tsp. Vitamin E*
- *1/4 tsp. modified lecithin*
- *1/4 tsp. evening primrose oil*
- *4 drops rose absolute*
- *4 drops jasmine absolute*

Mix all ingredients together and spoon into a sterile glass jar. Apply as needed.

To modify the recipe to suit normal to oily skin types, replace the jasmine and rose absolutes with twelve drops of essential oil of neroli, and replace the Vitamin E with Vitamin C. Apply as needed.

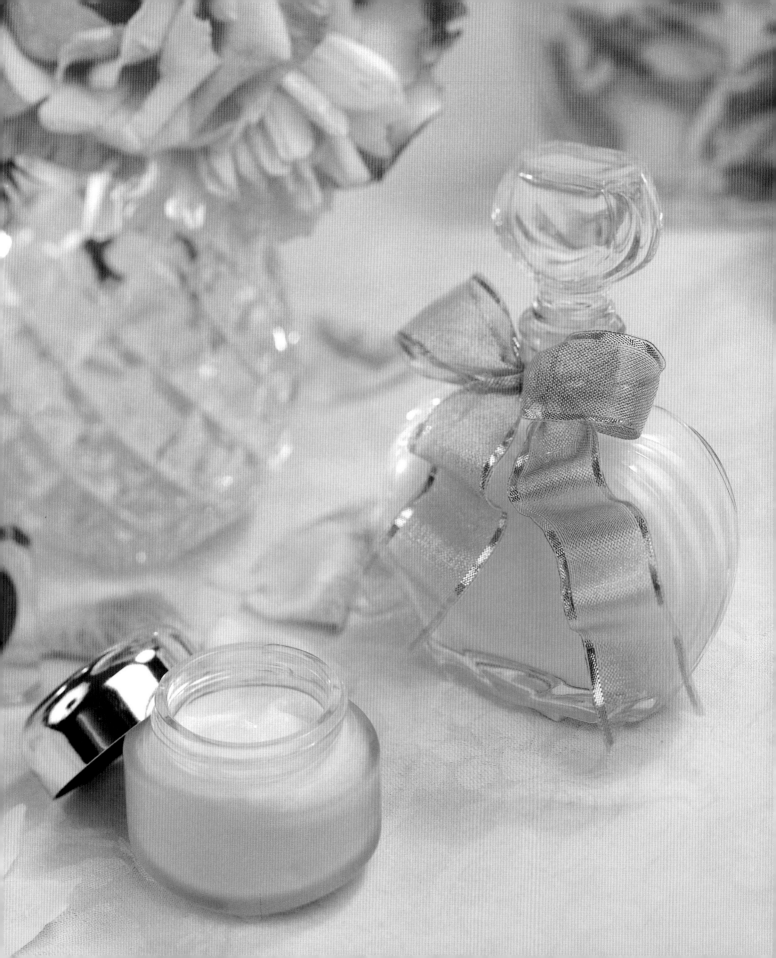

Specialty Oil Treatments

Specialty botanical oils are the central ingredients in these formulas, which have been created especially for dry, mature, sun-damaged skin, and for post-surgical recovery and skin repair. For many, the concept of massaging oils into facial skin for nourishment and skin regeneration is new and strange. The principal ingredient in many commercial oils and lotions is mineral oil, derived from hydrocarbons (petroleum.) Mineral oil has a large molecular structure which gives it good properties as a barrier for skin against the elements, but for other uses, it has a sticky, uncomfortable feel because it creates a layer over the pores, preventing skin cells from properly utilizing oxygen and nutrients. In recent studies, mineral oil has been shown to leach vitamins from the body. Once you become familiar with the wide variety of cold-pressed oils from botanical sources, you will be amazed at their nourishing and healing powers.

The best oils for facial skincare are fresh, cold-pressed oils from vegetable, seed and nut sources. Cold-pressing means that the oils are extracted without the use of excess heat, solvents or other refining chemicals or additives. Cold-pressed oils retain their full complement of essential fatty acids, vitamins and minerals, and each oil has slightly different properties. For example, oils such as sweet almond and apricot kernel are fine-textured, neutral oils, excellent for face and bodycare, while oils like jojoba or avocado are heavier, thicker oils which are better suited to hair and scalp treatments. Specialty oils such as wheatgerm, borage, evening primrose and vitamins A and E add exceptional nutrient value to all your facial skincare recipes.

PRECIOUS ESSENCE GOLDEN FACIAL OIL

An exceptional facial oil containing special botanical ingredients to nourish and rejuvenate face and neck. For all skin types.

- *2 tsp. (10 ml.) hazelnut oil*
- *2 tsp. (10 ml.) sweet almond oil*
- *1 tsp. (5 ml.) evening primrose oil*
- *1/2 tsp. (2.5 ml.) wheat germ oil*
- *10 drops Vitamin A*
- *10 drops Vitamin E*
- *10 drops sweet orange PEO*
- *10 drops sandalwood PEO*
- *5 drops frankincense PEO*
- *5 drops ylang-ylang PEO*
- *3 drops jasmine absolute (optional)*

Mix all ingredients together in a small beaker, and pour into a glass bottle (one with a built-in dropper is ideal.) Be sure your skin is clean and dry before applying the facial oil. Place a few drops on clean fingertips, and massage into the skin, using gentle but firm circular motions, concentrating on sensitive points on the face. Use the facial oil as often as desired, and add more if your skin absorbs it all.

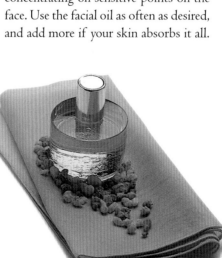

Many of the specialty oils have shown great potential in skin repair and regeneration, softening scar tissue, stimulating cell turnover and encouraging the rapid growth and development of healthy skin cells. This is due to the high content of anti-oxidant compounds and essential fatty acids as well as other skin-nourishing factors. Pure essential oils and oleoresins also exhibit remarkable antibacterial and preservative properties. Frankincense, myrrh and sandalwood were used in ancient Egypt to embalm and preserve the bodies of Pharaohs. When unearthed in the early twentieth century, many of the mummies showed no signs of deterioration!

SKIN REPAIR AND REGENERATION OIL

This formula is designed for special care of skin under stress from trauma such as surgery, scarring, sun damage and other environmental hazards.

- *3 tsp. (15 ml.) wheatgerm oil*
- *1 tsp. (5 ml.) evening primrose oil*
- *1 tsp. (5 ml.) calendula oil*
- *1/2 tsp. (2.5 ml.) Vitamin E*
- *8 drops frankincense PEO*
- *8 drops myrrh PEO*
- *8 drops sandalwood PEO*
- *3 drops benzoin oleoresin*
- *3 drops patchouli PEO*

Mix all ingredients together in a small beaker, stir well and pour into a glass bottle with built-in dropper. Apply to the affected area with clean fingertips and massage in gently, using circular motions, and concentrating on areas needing special care. Use the facial oil as often as needed, and repeat a second time if desired.

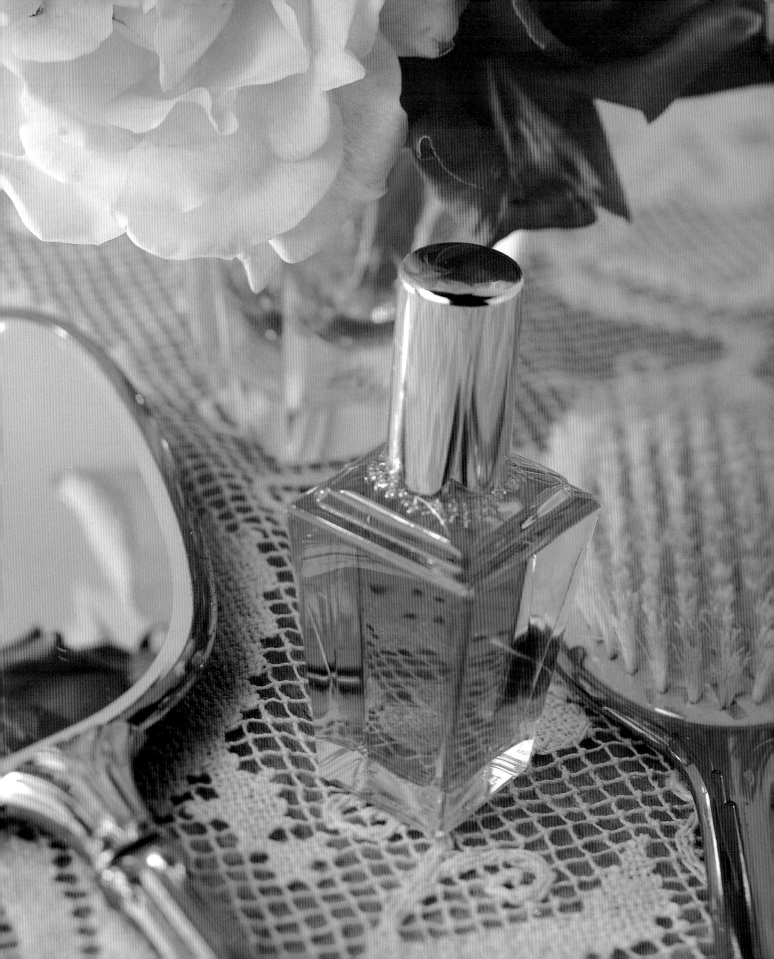

Chapter Six
Natural Bodycare

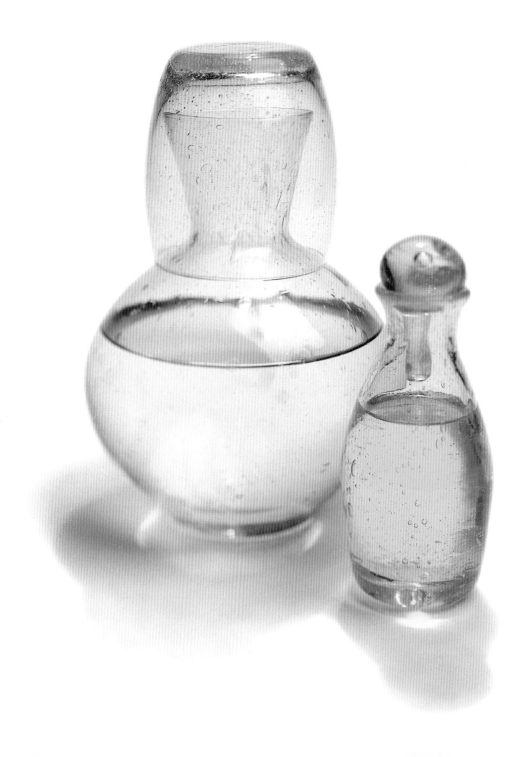

Introduction to Natural Bodycare

Throughout history, people from all countries and cultures have developed elaborate rituals for bathing, cleansing and beautifying the body. For centuries, the materials available for this purpose were all natural — water, clays, minerals, basic soaps, foodstuffs, herbs, oils, fats and aromatic materials from botanical sources. Trial and error ruled at first — even the discovery of soap came about through observation and experience. People noticed that bubbles were forming in rivers below animal sacrifice sites, a result of rain falling on the wood ashes and animal fats, creating a substance which proved good at removing dirt from the body. The oils of nuts and seeds when crushed for cooking were found to have softening, emollient properties on the skin. Herbs, trees and flowering plants were studied for their benefits, and people learned to make infused oils, salves and perfumes. Many of these bodycare recipes were so popular that they were recorded by the heads of the household for the use of future generations of family members, and these customized recipes (called 'receipts') were often closely guarded secrets. Increasingly, people who did not have access to the ministrations of physicians began to create their own homemade health and beauty preparations.

By the beginning of the twentieth century, the increase in the world's population and the onset of the scientific era had caused radical changes in the way medicine, health, beauty and household products were being formulated and manufactured. With the advent of technology, many natural ingredients which had proved their benefits over the course of centuries were ignored in favor of new chemical materials. In this new 'petroleum age,' products made with synthetic coal tar derivatives flooded the market. Mineral oil, detergents, dyes and synthetic fragrance 'aroma-chemicals' became commonplace, all derived from the relatively cheap, consistent supply of fossil fuel. Many people today do not realize that their bottle of fruit- or flower-flavored bath gel or expensive French perfume is derived from almost completely synthetic sources. Yet increasing problems from the constant use of these non-natural products is creating a growing demand for a return to simpler, more natural health and beauty products. Simplicity is not the only quality of Nature's offerings. Many of the same plant materials which were overlooked by scientists in the early days of cosmetic formulation are now being closely studied for their highly sophisticated structures and individual ingredients which are

of intense interest for medicinal and cosmetic research. Every day, new natural ingredients indigenous to many countries are being added to this list.

The recipes included in this section address many needs and include ingredients from basic, everyday materials to exotic, sophisticated new discoveries. On one end of the spectrum are fresh or dried herbs, which have been used for millenia, and on the other, pure essential oils (often from the very same plants) which were not available commercially until very recently. One of the pastimes where natural ingredients can be fully experienced and appreciated is bathing. Included are recipes for bathing with herbs, flowers, healing grains, sea salts, milk and other 'kitchen cosmetics,' infusions, oils, natural soaps and pure essential oils. Whether you're bathing to cleanse your body, relax your mind or soothe your soul, and more, you'll find formulas here to enjoy. The following pages will inspire you to create your own customized bath preparations as well.

Spa treatments are a specialized extension of natural bodycare. Salt glow rubs, full-body masks and scrubs, aromatherapy massage oils and specialized treatments using exotic natural materials are wonderful for both the body and the mind. While visiting a luxury spa is one of life's special treats, you can learn to make many of these healthful and beautifying recipes at home. Also included are recipes for products we use everyday — lotions, gels, powders, creams and perfumes. The difference is that these formulas are natural and omit the many problematic ingredients that are present in mass-produced cosmetic formulations. Using safe, nourishing ingredients from Nature, you can create, modify and customize these recipes. As you become familiar with natural ingredients and see the great improvement in your own well-being from using them, you'll be inspired to share your knowledge and creativity with your family and friends. Imagine surprising a special friend or relative with a custom body oil, lotion or aromatic splash that you have made yourself, designed just for them! Gift baskets of your natural bodycare products, designed to any theme you choose, are perfect for birthdays, anniversaries, holidays — virtually every occasion. Your personalized gift is sure to be remembered with special fondness for many years! Best of all, you'll be sharing the most important gift — Nature's vital essences for health and well-being, imbued with your own positive creativity and spirit.

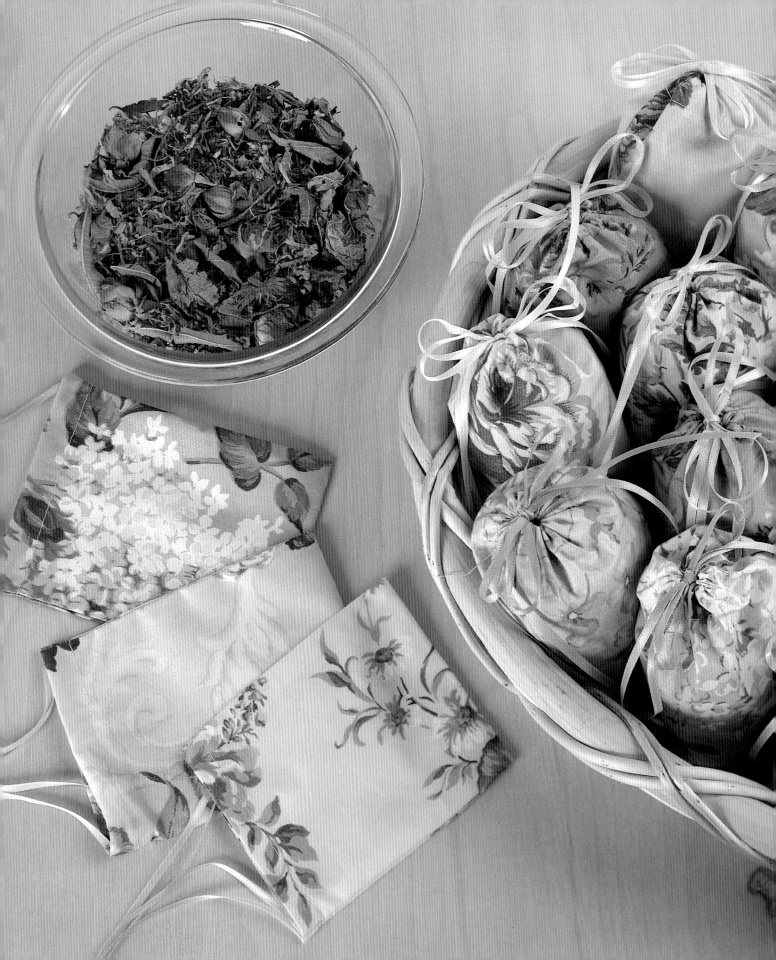

Herb and Flower Bath Sachets

Fragrant herb-filled sachets are a simple, old world way to enjoy the bounty of Nature, right out of your own herb or flower garden. Fresh or dried herbs and flowers provide us with true aromatherapy in its most elemental form. Envision rustic country houses, their heavy wooden beams adorned with abundant bunches of sweet-smelling field flowers, herbs, grasses and seedpods. Summer's colorful flower bouquets mingle with the brilliant green of culinary herbs and the lush beauty of harvest's treasures. If you have ever had the good fortune of visiting a place where herbs and flowers are drying naturally, you'll recall how the colors, textures and aromas of the scene uplifted and inspired you, providing pleasurable memories for the years to come. Preserve those memories by making your own natural potpourris, bath sachets and 'sweet bags' for use at home.

While herbal sachets for bathing and inhaling may seem quaint and old-fashioned, the aromatic pleasures they offer are very valuable in our stress-filled times. Imagine, for instance, sinking into a warm tub infused with the properties of fragrant botanicals, inhaling the soft, mind-clearing vapors, or sniffing an herbal sachet to alleviate a pounding headache or to lull you gently to sleep. One of the joys of collecting dried flowers and herbs is the adventure of creating naturally fragrant potpourris, herbal sleep pillows, drawer sachets, 'sweet bags,' relaxing eye pillows, soothing teas and bath infusions. To use in the bath, gather the dried materials together and fill and tie a pretty bag. The bath bag can be used several times if air-dried between uses, and can be turned inside out to be filled with new herbs and re-tied. Close the bathroom door, dim the lights, slip into the warm, fragrant water and let all your cares float away…

BOTANICAL TUB TEA

Delicious herbs and spices turn this bath into a healthy herbal brew! A great warming bath to ease the discomforts of the flu season.

- *2 Tbsp. rose petals*
- *2 Tbsp. rose geranium leaves*
- *1 Tbsp. rosemary leaves*
- *1 Tbsp. dried orange peel*
- *1" slice ginger root, chopped*
- *8 large clove buds*
- *1 tsp. powdered cinnamon*

Combine the dried herbs and spices and pile onto a 12" square piece of light cotton cloth. Sprinkle the cinnamon over the herbs. Tie up all four corners of the cloth, making a tight bundle. Toss the sachet in the hot running bathwater and let it infuse. As you take your bath, squeeze the bundle frequently to release its properties into the water — no soap is necessary. Inhale the rising vapors as you lie back and relax. After your bath, your body will feel aromatically cleansed, and you'll have renewed clarity and energy.

COUNTRY GARDEN BATH HERBS

An aromatic combination of herbs and flowers which have been used for centuries for their fragrant and healing benefits. This herb combination can be used for bath bags, drawer sachets and natural potpourris.

- *2 Tbsp. rose petals*
- *2 Tbsp. lavender flowers*
- *2 Tbsp. chamomile flowers*
- *2 Tbsp. peppermint leaves*
- *2 Tbsp. linden leaves*
- *2 Tbsp. lemongrass*

Gently combine the dried herbs and flowers in a bowl. To intensify the natural fragrance and create an aromatherapy effect, sprinkle a total of 30 drops of essential oils over the dried herbs, choosing from essential oils like geranium, lavender, lemongrass, palmarosa and ylang-ylang. Stir the herbs gently with a wooden spoon, and tuck the mixture into little fabric bags and tie shut. While your bath is pouring, drop the bag in the water and squeeze it several times to release the properties of the herbs and essential oils. Hold the filled sachet like a sponge in your hand, and rub it over your skin as you bathe to give it a soft and fragrant feel.

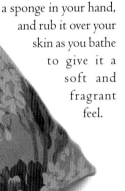

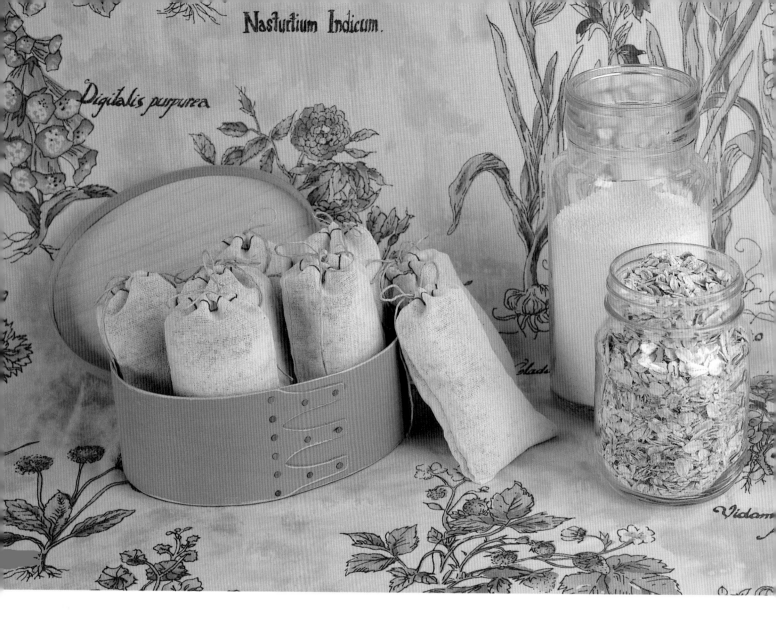

INGREDIENTS FOR MAKING THERAPEUTIC BATH BAGS, BY SKIN TYPE

For dry, sensitive or easily irritated skin:

- *fine-ground oatmeal*
- *almond meal and other nut meals*
- *powdered milk*
- *honey*
- *essential oils, e.g., lavender, rose geranium, chamomile, sandalwood, ylang-ylang*

For normal to dry skin:

- *oatmeal*
- *cornmeal*
- *almond meal*
- *dried citrus peel*
- *powdered herbs, e.g., benzoin, frankincense, myrrh, sandalwood*
- *essential oils, e.g., ylang-ylang, mandarin, sweet orange, lavender*

For oily, problem skin:

- *oatmeal*
- *cornmeal*
- *brans, e.g., oat, wheat and rice bran*
- *powdered herbs, e.g., goldenseal, echinacea, St. John's Wort*
- *essential oils, e.g., eucalyptus, lemon, rosemary, clary sage*

For itchy skin prone to rashes:

- *rice starch*
- *oat starch*
- *colloidal oatmeal*
- *powdered milk*
- *whey powder*
- *aloe vera powder*
- *honey*
- *essential oils, e.g., rose absolute, lavender, chamomile*

Therapeutic Bath Sachets

Soaking in a tub of warm fragrant water is one of the most relaxing, effective ways of reducing stress as well as giving yourself a full-body skincare treatment. If you have dry, dehydrated skin, or if you are prone to allergies, rashes and other skin irritations, you can make healing bath sachets using ingredients you probably have right in your kitchen! Simple, natural ingredients like oatmeal, ground grain and nut meals and brans, honey and milk provide much-needed nourishment to troubled skin, and bathwater makes the perfect carrier to disperse these healing agents.

Oatmeal in particular has a long tradition of regulating and balancing the skin and assisting in skin metabolism. Cultivated cereal oats (Avena sativa) are rich in vitamins, minerals and amino acids, as well as beta glucan, a natural humectant capable of penetrating the skin to moisturize and nourish. The unique composition of nutrients in oatmeal gives it its special ability to relieve itching and inflammation and its remarkable cleansing and skin-soothing abilities when added to bathwater. Colloidal oatmeal is routinely prescribed by doctors for a variety of skin disorders including hives, eczema, psoriasis, sunburn, insect bites and skin rashes. In addition to oatmeal, ground nut and grain meals and brans are natural substances that soothe inflamed, rough or itchy skin. Almond meals and other finely-ground nut meals are full of vitamins and natural oils. Oat bran, wheat bran and rice bran add a gentle bio-active exfoliating element to bath bags. Powdered milk contains protein, calcium and vitamins. You can easily make your own therapeutic bath bags at home by combining grain meals with powdered herbs and essential oils.

First, select your ingredients from the list opposite, and combine the meals, starches or brans in a bowl. If you are treating a specific skin condition, stir in herbal powders and essential oils next. Stir constantly as you add essential oils drop by drop. When the mixture is fully blended, fill small unbleached muslin bags with the mixture. The loose weave of the muslin fabric will enable the ingredients inside to infuse the bathwater with their healing powers. Place a bath bag under the faucet and pour your bath. You'll notice the water turning a creamy, opaque color, with a texture like silk. While bathing, hold the bag in your hand and rub it all over your body. No soap is needed for this special bath treatment — the ingredients are natural cleansers that draw dirt and oils away from the skin. If you haven't taken a bath using these therapeutic ingredients before, you'll be surprised by the soft, velvety feel of your skin as it absorbs nutrients from the bag and the bathwater.

OAT AND MILK SACHETS WITH YLANG-YLANG

Aromatic bath bags that soothe irritated skin while imparting the sweet fragrance of tropical flowers. For all skin types.

- *6 Tbsp. ground oatmeal*
- *6 Tbsp. powdered milk*
- *30 drops ylang-ylang PEO*

Combine the ingredients thoroughly and fill small bath bags. Tie bags tightly, and store in a dry place. Use as needed.

NOURISHING CITRUS ALMOND SACHETS

A delicious mixture of skin-smoothing ingredients to clarify and nurture problem skin. For all skin types.

- *4 Tbsp. oatmeal*
- *4 Tbsp. ground almond meal*
- *1 Tbsp. powdered milk*
- *1 Tbsp. dried orange peel*
- *1 Tbsp. sandalwood powder*
- *1 Tbsp. unpasteurized honey*
- *30 drops sweet orange PEO*

Combine all ingredients in a bowl, stirring well. Stuff the mixture into muslin bags, tie and store. Use as needed.

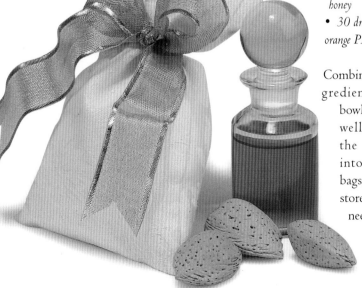

Mineral Bath Salts

For centuries, people the world over have known about the therapeutic power of bathing in water rich in minerals. Minerals and trace elements deep-cleanse and revitalize the body and help it maintain its regular functions. In countries around the globe, hot springs and mineral bath resorts feature waters with their own unique mineral composition. In Germany, the famed 'Kurbad' ('cure-bath') of Baden-Baden offers potent mineral water and invigorating pine-scented air to visitors 'taking the cure.' Resorts in France and Italy offer mineral baths with benefits to those suffering from arthritis, heart disease, muscular and circulatory disorders and skin conditions. The Dead Sea in Israel is another area that attracts thousands of visitors a year. One of the lowest points on earth, the Dead Sea contains a high percentage of natural minerals proven to be extremely helpful in the treatment of skin conditions like eczema and psoriasis. Many conditions pronounced 'incurable' have shown marked improvement or even resolved completely after mineral hydrotherapy treatments.

Other forms of water therapy are seawater bathing ('balneotherapy') and the use of mineral-rich seaweeds and algae in bodycare formulations ('thalassotherapy.') Mineral-rich sea salts make an excellent carrier base for dried herbs, herb powders and essential oils, so that you can customize your bath salt recipes. When selecting salts for your bathing formulas, be sure to select natural, untreated salts, such as the solar-dried sea salts from New Zealand (available in coarse or fine grades,) the moist greyish natural sea salts from the French coast, or potent Dead Sea mineral salts. You can also add Epsom salts (magnesium sulfate) for muscle aches and pains, or sodium bicarbonate for a refreshing fizzy effect. Table salt (sodium chloride) is often treated with an additive to keep it free-flowing. Avoid this if you can, and concentrate on obtaining mineral-rich natural salts. Mix them in a glass or ceramic bowl using wooden utensils (avoid contact with metals,) and store your customized salts in airtight glass containers away from excessive heat, light or moisture.

SPRINGTIME LAVENDER MINERAL BATH SALTS

The clean, fresh aroma of lavender is always a welcome addition to a bath, particularly in addition to toning and purifying mineral salts. For all skin types.

- *1/2 cup (4 oz.) solar-dried sea salts*
- *1/4 cup (2 oz.) Epsom salts*
- *1/4 cup (2 oz.) Dead Sea mineral salts*
- *40 drops lavender PEO*

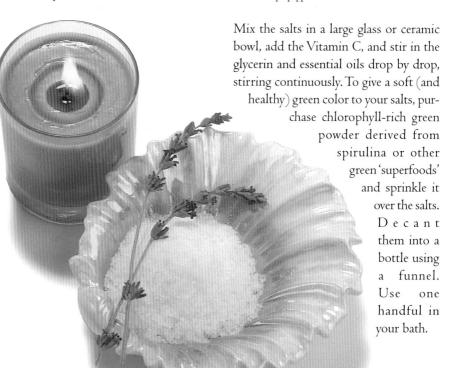

Mix all the ingredients together in a large bowl and stir until well blended. This recipe yields crisp, snow-white bath salts with a wonderful fragrance. Store in a glass bottle and use one handful to a bath.

SEA FOAM MINERAL BATH SALTS WITH PEPPERMINT

These cleansing salts combine with the fresh, clean fragrance of peppermint and rosemary to stimulate and energize the body. Rosemary, from the Latin 'ros marinus,' literally means 'dew of the sea.' These salts look beautiful displayed in a large glass decanter in the bathroom. For all skin types.

- *2 cups (16 oz.) solar-dried sea salts*
- *1/4 cup (2 oz.) Dead Sea mineral salts*
- *1/4 cup (2 oz.) sodium bicarbonate*
- *1 Tbsp. vegetable glycerin*
- *1 tsp. Vitamin C powder*
- *50 drops rosemary PEO*
- *50 drops peppermint PEO*

Mix the salts in a large glass or ceramic bowl, add the Vitamin C, and stir in the glycerin and essential oils drop by drop, stirring continuously. To give a soft (and healthy) green color to your salts, purchase chlorophyll-rich green powder derived from spirulina or other green 'superfoods' and sprinkle it over the salts. Decant them into a bottle using a funnel. Use one handful in your bath.

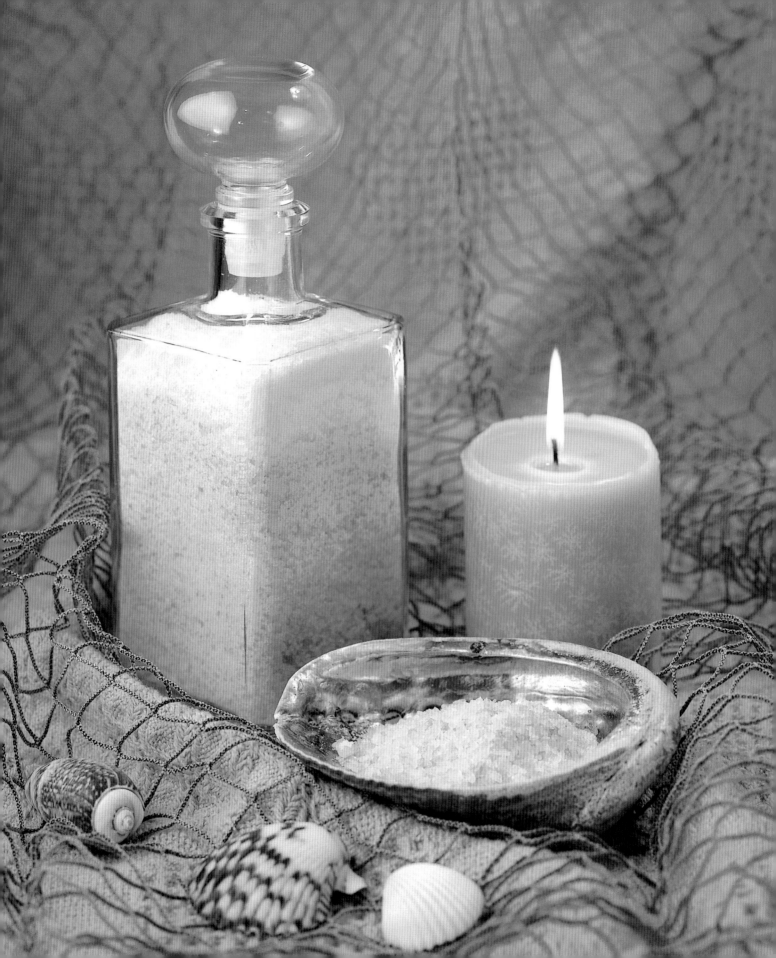

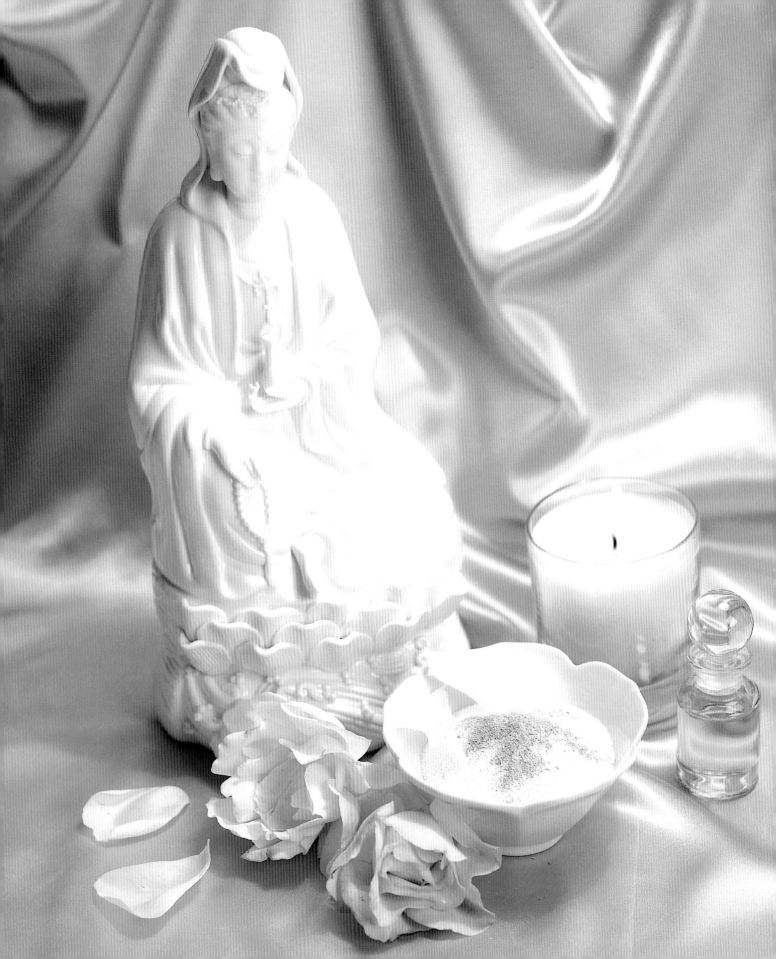

Milk Baths

Everyone knows the story of Cleopatra and her legendary aromatic milk baths, to which she attributed her renowned powers of charm and seduction. Milk baths are a mainstay in beauty folklore, with famous beauties through the ages testifying to their youth-enhancing, revitalizing properties. Poppea, the wife of Emperor Nero, bathed in asses' milk, while Marie Antoinette's favorite wrinkle preventive was buttermilk. The famous French beauty Ninon de l'Enclos was reputedly attracting young lovers right up to the time of her death at the age of ninety-one. Her secret was her famed beauty mask, made of boiled milk, lemon juice and brandy, which she applied each night and morning. Colonial ladies, perhaps following her example, were said to have combined milk and whiskey for a skin-cleansing beauty treatment.

The reasons for milk's great popularity lie in its excellent nutritive value in skincare. Milk is packed with proteins, beneficial fats, vitamins, amino acids and calcium, and is readily absorbed by the skin, resulting in a smooth, hydrated appearance. A simple way of experiencing milk's benefits is to pour a pint of regular milk into your bath, stir, and soak for 10 – 15 minutes. Your skin will be noticeably softer and smoother, with a dewy sheen. Milk is also an excellent carrier for essential oils, dispersing the molecules thoroughly through the bathwater. You can use 10 - 12 drops of essential oil (or oil blend) of your choice in 8 ounces of milk. For dryer skin types, use milk with a higher butterfat content, including whole milk, half-and-half, and cream. For oilier skin types, use skim milk, low-fat milk, or powdered milk.

EVERYDAY MILK BATH

The nutritive values of milk combine with the therapeutic values of essential oils to create a fragrant and relaxing bathing experience. You can vary the essential oils used depending on the aromatherapeutic effect you wish to achieve.

- *8 oz. (240 ml.) whole milk*
- *10 drops sweet orange PEO*

The soft citrusy aroma of this bath makes it a favorite at any time of day. Combine the ingredients, and stir into bathwater. Soak for 10 – 15 minutes.

ROSE PETAL MILK BATH

An aromatic treat for a special occasion! A soft, silky bath that feels like a bed of roses. For all skin types.

- *1 cup (8 oz.) powdered milk*
- *handful red rose petals, dried*
- *40 drops rose geranium PEO*
- *rose absolute (optional)*

Place drops of essential oil or absolute on each rose petal. Mix the petals gently into the milk powder, and pour into a decorative decanter. Use a handful in each bath.

Vary floral milk baths by using jasmine flowers, orange blossoms, lavender buds, lemon verbena, or other dried flowers or herbs from your garden.

KWAN YIN SERENITY BATH

Subtle spice, fruit and flower aromas combine with nutrient-rich milk to create a sensual, euphoric bathing experience. For all skin types.

- *1 cup (8 oz.) powdered milk*
- *1 Tbsp. Chinese five spice mixture*
- *20 drops mandarin PEO*
- *10 drops sandalwood PEO*
- *10 drops ylang-ylang PEO*

Combine the ingredients in a bowl, stir well, and store in an airtight glass jar. Use a handful in each bath. Relax and dream awhile!

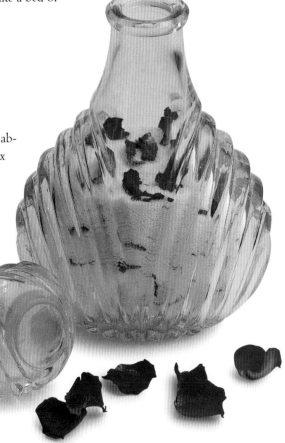

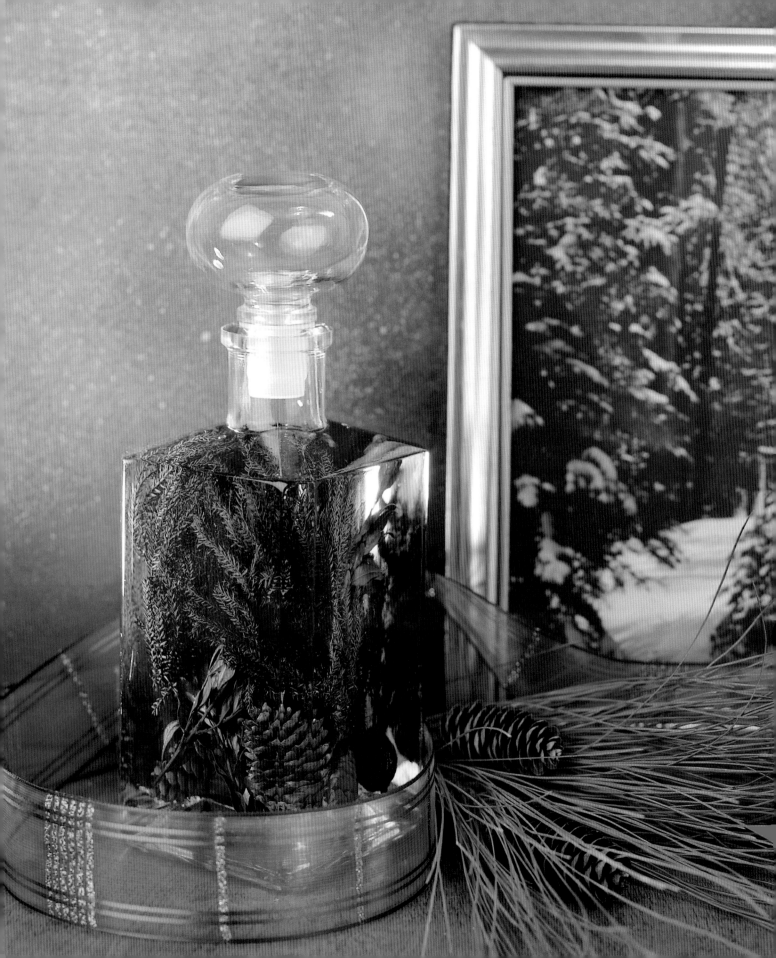

Bath Oils

The concept of 'bath oil' is currently undergoing a radical change. Today's aromatherapeutic bath oils have literally nothing in common with the artificially-scented, mineral oil-based products typically found in the department store or drugstore. Realizing that bathing is one of the major ways of treating the skin of the entire body to beneficial nutrients suspended in the bathwater, progressive product manufacturers are formulating a new generation of healing bath oils. These formulas contain the latest ingredients proven to have excellent skin-repairing qualities, such as cold-pressed plant oils, phospholipids, vitamins, herbal oils and essential oils. If your skin has a tendency towards dryness, itchiness or flaking, natural bath oils will provide superior moisturizing qualities that will quickly eliminate these problems.

At the forefront of research into skin repair substances are essential fatty acids, found in cold-pressed plant oils, and phosphatidylcholine, found in soybean lecithin. Together with essential oils, these substances have the ability to smooth skin and help it function optimally. Prepare the basic recipe given in Chapter Three, and add essential oils to suit your mood and skincare needs. Herbal oils are balancing and therapeutic; citrus and spice oils are comforting and warming; floral and woodsy oils are relaxing and euphoric. Unlike traditional bath oil, natural bath oils do not have a greasy feel, and it is easy to clean the tub after using them. This is due to the phospholipids, which are natural emulsifiers. These compounds have a natural affinity for the skin, and will begin their skin repair and nourishing functions as soon as you submerge yourself in the bath.

To use natural bath oils effectively, run your bath and when it is almost full, pour 1 – 2 Tbsp. of the oil into the water. Soak in the tub for 15 – 20 minutes, running your hands through the water and massaging the beneficial oils into your skin. After your bath, pat yourself dry with a towel. Your skin will feel renewed — even-textured, baby-soft and silky. Note: if you have been physically active prior to bathing, it is recommended that you take a quick hot shower beforehand to remove excess dirt and sweat. The oils in these formulas create an effective repair complex that works best on clean skin.

INVIGORATING BAVARIAN PINE BATH OIL

Inspired by the pine forests of Bavaria, this intensely aromatic bath oil deep-cleanses and detoxifies both the skin and the lungs. Once you are in the bath, breathe deeply to take full advantage of the aromatherapeutic vapors rising from the tub, while the oils smooth and nourish your skin.

- *8 oz. (240 ml.) unfragranced bath oil (see formula in Chapter Three)*
- *50 drops pine needle PEO*
- *10 drops sandalwood PEO*
- *10 drops cedarwood Atlas PEO*
- *10 drops pimento berry PEO*

Pour the unfragranced bath oil into a large beaker or measuring cup, and add the essential oils. Stir until thoroughly blended. Decant the oil into a decorative glass bottle and cap tightly. You can add dried pine cones and dried green conifer branches to create a "forest in a bottle." Keep the decanter away from bright light or excessive heat. The bottle can be refilled with bath oil at any time.

CITRUS BLOSSOM SMOOTHING BATH OIL

The soft and euphoric fragrance of real orange blossom combined with the skin-nourishing qualities of fresh natural oils.

- *8 oz. (240 ml.) unfragranced bath oil (see formula in Chapter Three)*
- *40 drops bitter orange PEO*
- *20 drops sweet orange PEO*
- *10 drops ylang-ylang PEO*
- *10 drops neroli PEO*

Pour the unfragranced bath oil into a large beaker or measuring cup, and add the essential oils. Stir until thoroughly blended. Decant the oil into a decorative glass bottle and cap. If desired, add dried orange peel and orange blossom to the bottle for a nice visual effect.

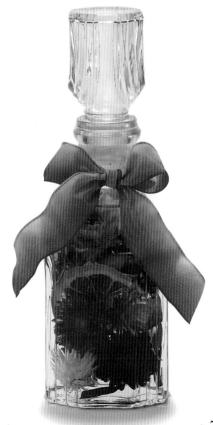

Bath and Shower Gels

Many of us remember scenes from Hollywood movies where the seductress reclines languidly in a bathtub filled with mounds of bubbles, a diamond-clad hand holding aloft a flute of sparkling champagne. Glamorous as such images were, the reality of bubble baths of the time was rather different. The earliest liquid soaps for bathing were highly effective cleansers, but they were so strong that many users soon developed itchy skin, eczema and dermatitis. In the 1960's, dermatological problems coupled with environmental pollution from these non-biodegradable detergent ingredients caused concerned citizens and the medical profession to demand changes in soap formulations.

Today, ingredient disclosures on bath and shower gels are invariably very similar. Serviceable synthetic surfactants, mostly coconut-derived cleansers that have been alkoxylated (created through chemical reaction with fatty alcohols, sulfuric acid and other ingredients) combined with synthetic emulsifiers, stabilizers and preservatives, form the basis for most soap gels. These gels are then artificially fragranced with aroma-chemicals and tinted with synthetic colors. Most ingredients used in this product category are cheap and readily available for cosmetic product formulation. However, the formulas themselves are far from natural, and do pose potential skin irritation hazards for a significant (and increasing) percentage of the population, particularly children and those with sensitive skin. Now you can create effective, skin-smoothing natural gels at home, adding the herbal infusions, essential oils and special bio-active ingredients of your choice. Formulas for two natural bases are

given in Chapter Three, and both easily accept botanical ingredients and keep them in suspension and active, ready for any aromatherapeutic bath or shower application.

JASMINE FLOWERS BATH AND SHOWER GEL

A mild gel for a bath full of soft bubbles with the exquisite, relaxing aroma of jasmine flowers. For all skin types.

- *8 oz. (240 ml.) unfragranced gel base (see Chapter Three)*
- *40 drops ylang-ylang PEO*
- *10 drops jasmine absolute*

Combine the ingredients in a beaker or measuring cup and stir thoroughly. Using a funnel, pour into a plastic squeeze bottle for easy use for shower or bath. Use with a sponge, loofah or washcloth for best results.

HEAVENLY CITRUS BATH AND SHOWER GEL

A sensory delight, combining citrus and floral oils for a dreamy bath experience. For all skin types.

- *8 oz. (240 ml.) unfragranced gel base (see Chapter Three)*
- *40 drops sweet orange PEO*
- *20 drops ylang-ylang PEO*
- *10 drops grapefruit PEO*
- *10 drops bergamot PEO*

Combine all ingredients in a measuring cup, stir well, and pour into a bottle. Use 1-2 Tbsp. for each bath or shower.

DEODORIZING HERBAL SHOWER GEL

A fresh, therapeutic gel to cleanse and deodorize skin, heal infections and stimulate skin cell regeneration. For all skin types.

- *4 oz. (120 ml.) unfragranced liquid coconut soap*
- *2 oz. (60 ml.) chamomile infusion*
- *2 oz. (60 ml.) aloe vera gel*
- *30 drops rosemary PEO*
- *20 drops lemon PEO*
- *20 drops lavender PEO*
- *10 drops white thyme PEO*

Mix all ingredients together, and pour into a plastic bottle with dispenser top. Use in the bath or shower with a loofah, mitt or sponge.

For extra anti-bacterial effect, add drops of the following pure essential oils to unfragranced gel:
- tea tree
- eucalyptus
- pine needle
- cajeput

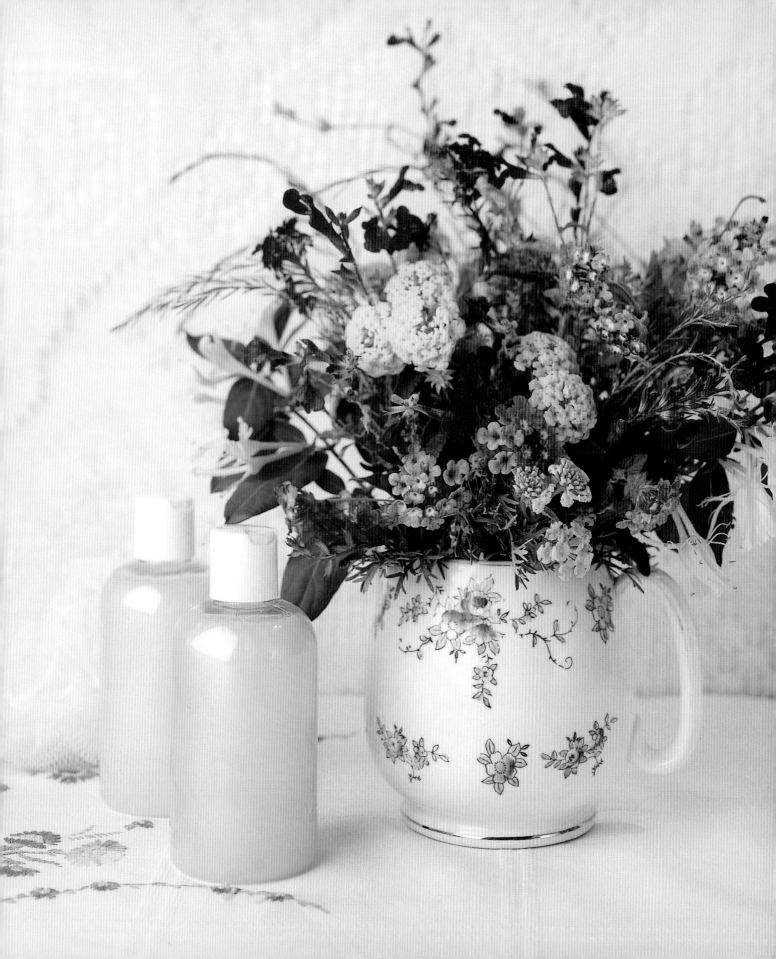

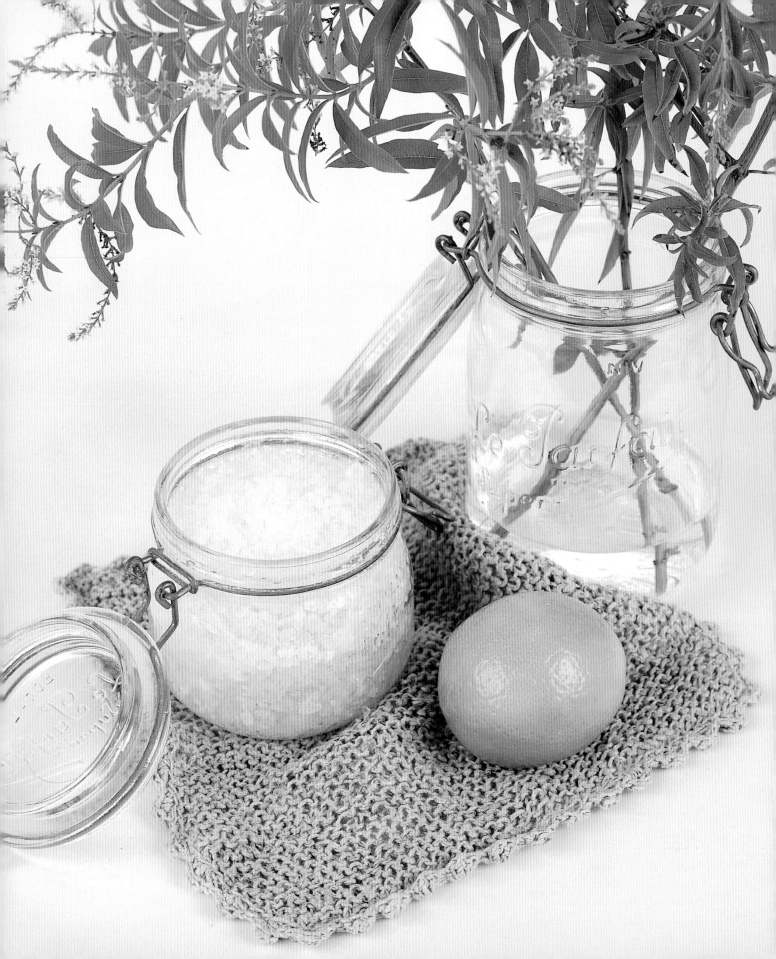

Body Scrubs

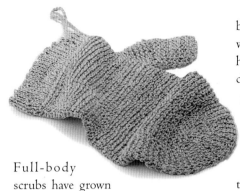

Full-body scrubs have grown in popularity in recent years. Spas the world over now offer a menu of body scrubs, ranging from 'salt glow' rubs to complex treatments using a variety of exotic oils, herbs, fibrous materials and powders. The simple 'salt glow' is a very effective skin exfoliant, deep-cleanser and detoxifier. In this treatment, natural sea salts are rubbed over dampened skin by a technician using hands or a special mitt. Then, once all the body skin has been treated, the spa guest is treated to full body skin brushing followed by an exhilarating shower and, since salts can have a slightly drying effect, a massage using natural body oil or lotion to replenish moisture. This treatment clears the skin of dead skin cells, encourages elimination of toxins and impurities through the pores, and brings a rosy, healthy glow to the renewed skin.

Most people are familiar with body scrub products sold in stores, in which gritty particles are held in suspension in a soapy, lotion-like base. If you would like to create a natural version of this type of product, it is possible to do so by combining fine-ground, dried plant-derived materials to the gel base described in Chapter Three. Typically, crushed black walnut, almond or apricot shells provide the exfoliating factor in scrubs. Bear in mind that, if not fine-ground, these can be quite gritty and are best suited to those with oilier, coarser skin. An excellent home replacement is raw, turbinado or demerara sugar, added to the gel base just prior to giving yourself a full-body scrub treatment. Other food-based scrubs and exfoliants like almond meal, herbal powders and fine-ground citrus peel can be added to the gel just before treatment. Use about 1 Tbsp. of scrub material to a full handful of gel base, or mix in a small bowl for convenience.

LEMON VERBENA SPA SALT GLOW

A superb refreshing and moisturizing allover body polish. This spa recipe combines purifying salts with cleansing essential oils and fine-textured almond oil for moisturizing and to give your skin a healthy, glowing finish.

* 1 cup (8 oz.) coarse sea salts
* 8 oz. (240 ml.) sweet almond oil
* 40 drops lemon PEO
* 20 drops lemon verbena PEO
* 20 drops grapefruit PEO
* 10 drops juniper berry PEO
* 10 drops ylang-ylang PEO

Stir the essential oils into the sweet almond oil in a measuring cup or beaker. Place the salts in a glass kitchen jar with gasket-type closure. Pour the oil mixture over the salts, close the jar, and let the oils soak into the salts. After several minutes, invert the jar so that the salts become more saturated. Turn the jar right side up one more time. To use, slip on a dampened hemp, cotton or natural mesh body mitt and take a handful of salts in your palm. Standing in the shower, use the mitt with the salts to give yourself a 3 – 5 minute all-over body treatment, using gentle circular motions. Add more salts as needed. Finish your session with a brisk, cool shower, and rub yourself dry with a clean towel. Your skin will feel invigorated and brand new!

VANILLA SUGAR BODY SCRUB

* 2 oz (60 ml.) unfragranced gel base (see Chapter Three)
* 1/2 oz. (15 ml.) vegetable glycerin
* 2 Tbsp. raw brown sugar
* 20 drops vanilla oleoresin
* 5 drops patchouli PEO
* 5 drops ylang-ylang PEO

Pour the gel base and glycerin into a small bowl, and add the sugar and essential oils. Rub mixture over your body with your hands or a mitt, using circular motions. Follow with a shower with the faucet turned full on. Towel dry and apply a light moisturizer. You will feel and smell delicious!

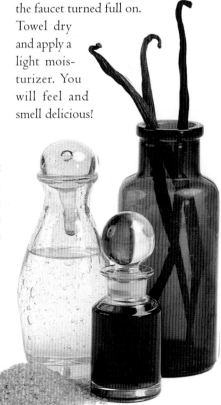

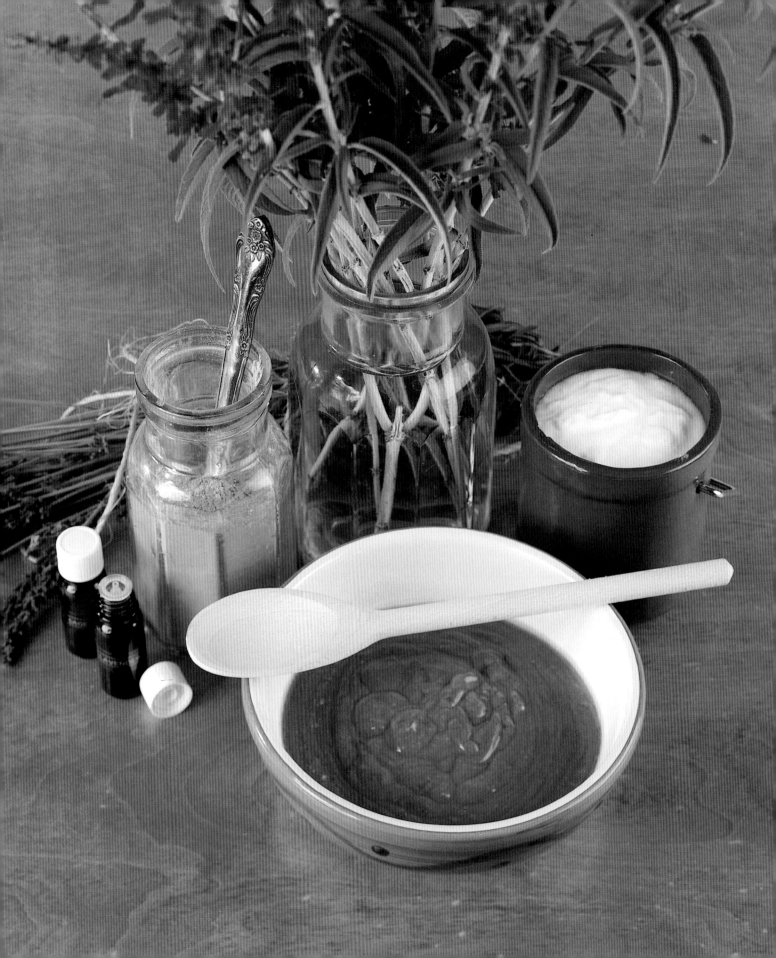

Body Masks

A long-time favorite at spas, full-body masks provide cleansing, detoxifying and rejuvenating benefits to skin. While we spend a lot of attention on facial skincare, body skin is often overlooked. Body skin deserves assistance in shedding flaky, dead skin cells, alleviating dry and rough patches, restoring moisture balance and encouraging a fresh, youthful appearance. Frequent dry brushing, scrubs, bathing and massages are a good adjunct to these full-body masks made with clays and other natural ingredients. Making a clay or mud body mask involves a little play therapy. Mixing and applying the squishy green mush brings out the child in just about everyone! Although you might look like the monster from the slimy depths for 20 minutes or so, the improvements to your skin tone and texture will be well worth the experience.

While clay and mud body masks suit normal to oily skin types, nourishing and moisturizing masks can also be made to improve dry or dehydrated skin. In place of clay, these body masks use honey, eggs, cream and other foods rich in vitamins, minerals and amino acids. Nutritive body treatments such as these cost a lot of money at luxury spas. Have fun creating your own at home! To get started, select a recipe and mix up enough for one session. Take a quick warm bath or shower. Then, using your hands or an inexpensive bristle paintbrush, cover yourself with the mask mixture from head to toe. Use an old sheet to cover a comfy place to lie down for 15 – 20 minutes while the mask dries. Then rinse off in the shower, first with warm water, then with cool. Pat yourself dry and see how soft and rejuvenated your skin feels!

LAVENDER AND SAGE PURIFYING CLAY BODY MASK

This body mask combines deep-cleansing, mineral-rich sea clay, live yogurt, honey and therapeutic essential oils of French lavender and Spanish sage to create a powerful 'spring cleaning' effect. Be sure to drink lots of cool mineral or spring water during and after this full-body treatment.

- *1/2 cup (4 oz.) sea clay powder*
- *1 cup (8 oz.) cultured, unflavored yogurt*
- *2 Tbsp. unpasteurized honey*
- *1 tsp. (5 ml.) evening primrose oil*
- *1/2 tsp. Vitamin E*
- *25 drops French lavender PEO*
- *25 drops Spanish sage PEO*

Mix the yogurt, honey, evening primrose oil, Vitamin E and essential oils together in a glass or ceramic bowl until thoroughly blended. Add the sea clay powder one teaspoon at a time until you reach the desired consistency for your skin type. Follow the directions given above for applying the body mask. After showering, dry your skin and apply a light moisturizer.

NOURISHING MILK AND HONEY BODY MASK

This nutritious mask uses raw unpasteurized honey and protein-rich milk and eggs. Fragrant essential oils, brandy, vanilla and vitamins give this body mask an exquisite rich aroma.

- *4 oz. (120 ml.) warmed honey*
- *2 oz. (60 ml.) cream*
- *1 egg*
- *1/2 oz. (15 ml.) brandy*
- *1/2 tsp. Vitamin E*
- *20 drops vanilla oleoresin*
- *20 drops bitter orange PEO*
- *10 drops ylang-ylang PEO*

Warm the honey by placing the uncapped glass jar in a pot of boiled water. Pour the honey into a glass bowl and add the other ingredients. When the mixture is smooth, apply to your skin with your hands or a paintbrush. Lie down and relax for 20-30 minutes, covering yourself with an old sheet or blanket to retain body heat while the ingredients moisturize and nourish. Afterwards, shower well and pat yourself dry with a towel.

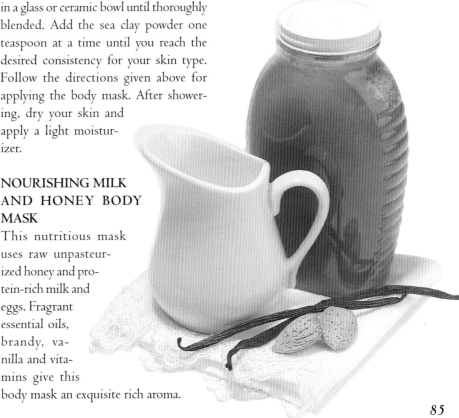

Cellulite Treatments

It is estimated that over 80% of women have some amount of cellulite, and while this distressing condition is most often associated with being overweight, it is also found among men and those who are underweight. While inactivity and hormonal causes are often attributed, the primary cause of cellulite is the constant ingestion of chemical additives, preservatives, and other non-nutritious components of the typical western diet. The body's lymphatic system, responsible for filtering toxins, deposits these substances in areas of the body away from the vital organs, namely, the hips, buttocks and thighs. Here, due to genetic, hormonal and structural considerations, the cellulite is manifested in the form of lumpy, rippled 'orange peel' skin that is often bloated and sensitive.

With dedication and perseverance, it is possible to rid the body of cellulite. A natural foods diet, aerobic and strength-training exercise, dry brushing, saunas, lymphatic and deep-tissue massage are a necessary part of any cellulite reduction program. Natural products containing bio-active herbal extracts and specific essential oils are also important. Traditional plant materials for fighting cellulite are ivy, horse chestnut, broom, horsetail, ginseng, sea algae and the mineral-rich seaweeds kelp and bladderwrack. Pure essential oils used in cellulite treatments include grapefruit, lemon, juniper berry, cypress and rosemary, all renowned for their diuretic and purifying effects. Dietary supplementation with specific nutrients including antioxidants and lipotropic factors is very helpful. Resolution of mental and emotional issues is also important and should be addressed with stress reduction techniques, meditation and creative visualization. If you are serious about eliminating cellulite, regular use of the cellulite-reduction formulas that follow will start you on the path to breaking free of this stubborn condition. For best results, seek out a sympathetic and knowledgeable natural health professional who is familiar with the causes and treatment of cellulite, and take advantage of the many avenues which exist to eliminate this obstacle to total mind/body health and wellness.

IVY AND GRAPEFRUIT BODY SCRUB

The common garden plant, ivy (Hedera helix) contains phyto-factors that are considered to be excellent in cellulite reduction. Grapefruit and juniper berry essential oils are diuretic and detoxifying, and complement the other ingredients in the formula.

- *6 oz. (180 ml.) unfragranced gel (see Chapter Three)*
- *1 1/2 oz. (45 ml.) ivy extract*
- *4 Tbsp. black walnut hulls*
- *60 drops grapefruit PEO*
- *30 drops juniper berry PEO*
- *15 drops bitter orange PEO*
- *15 drops cypress PEO*

Pour the gel and ivy extract into a measuring cup or beaker. Stir with a spoon or rod and add the essential oils, stirring well until completely blended. Using a funnel, pour the mixture into an 8 oz. plastic bottle. Before giving yourself a treatment, add 1 Tbsp. black walnut hulls to 1 - 2 oz. gel in a small bowl. Massage the gel over your body daily while showering using a loofah, cloth or body mitt.

IVY AND GRAPEFRUIT BODY LOTION

After showering or bathing, this cellulite fighter supplies plant-derived active ingredients to detoxify and tone body skin.

- *6 oz. (180 ml.) unfragranced body lotion (see Chapter Three)*
- *1 1/2 oz. (45 ml.) ivy extract*
- *1 Tbsp. (30 ml.) unflavored vodka*
- *1 Tbsp (30 ml.) vegetable glycerin*
- *60 drops grapefruit PEO*
- *30 drops juniper berry PEO*
- *15 drops bitter orange PEO*
- *15 drops cypress PEO*

Pour all ingredients into a glass bowl, stir, and when blended, pour into an 8 oz. bottle. Apply the lotion liberally after showering. When applying, use the palms of the hands and the fingertips to massage the cellulite-affected areas with a kneading motion. Press deeply and firmly to loosen excess fluids and toxins from the muscle tissues. Finish with long smoothing motions with the palms. Let the lotion sink into the skin, and towel off later if desired. Use the gel and lotion as often as desired for best results.

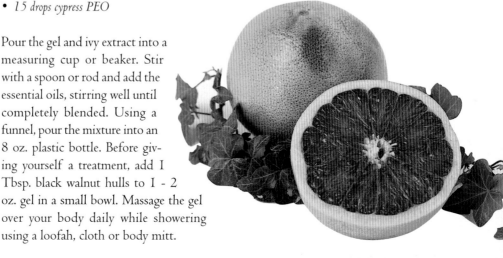

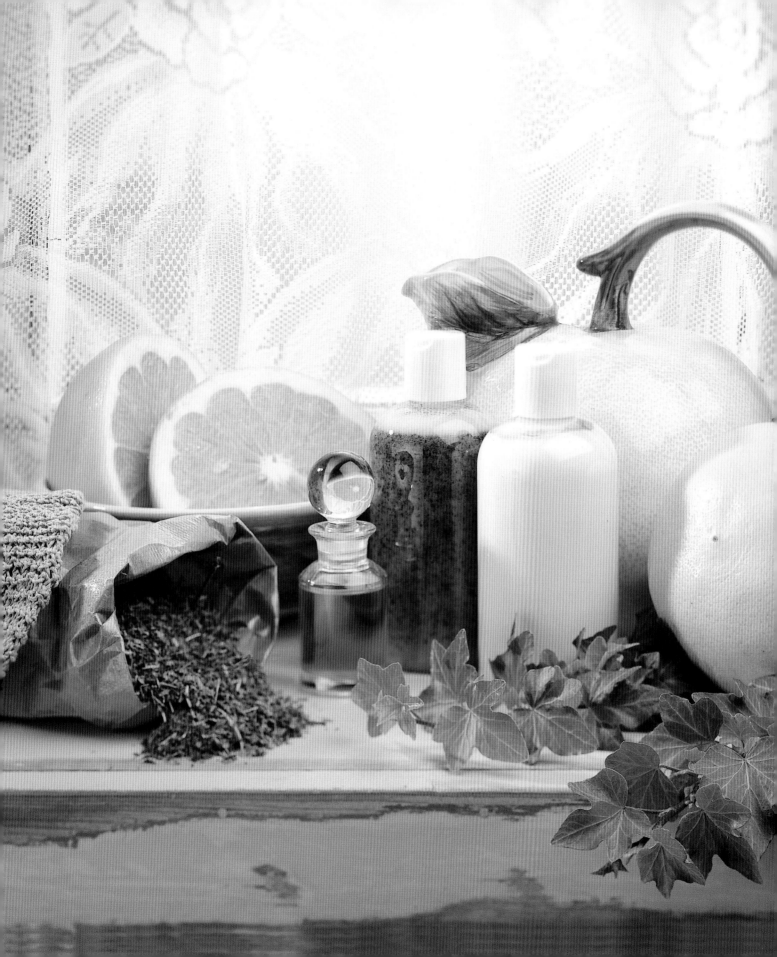

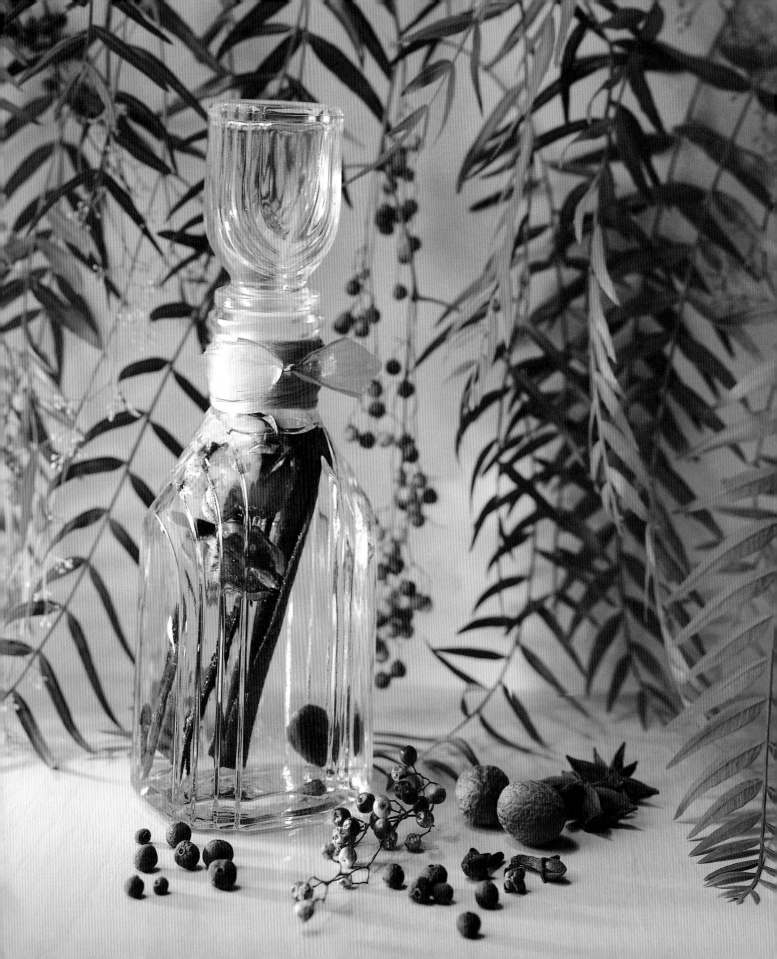

Body Splashes and Tonics

Naturally aromatic body splashes are simple to make, and are milder for your skin than their commercial counterparts, with much less likelihood of sensitivity or irritation. You can make great early morning wake-up refreshers, cooling spritzers for a muggy summer day, or reviving splashes for use after the bath or before a big night out. The advantage of natural homemade splashes over commercial products lies in the ingredients. Most commercial splashes and colognes contain a high percentage of SD ('Special Denatured') alcohol, so called because poisonous substances have been added to make it undrinkable. Commercial splashes also contain synthetic scents and colors which pose problems for those with skin sensitivities or allergies.

When making your own body splashes and tonics, you can decide how astringent or mild you would like the formula to be. Mild formulas contain high percentages of spring water or mineral water with the addition of pure aloe vera gel and vegetable glycerin. Bracing toners contain witch hazel extract, an herbal distillate containing 14 % alcohol, or a pure drinking alcohol like unflavored vodka. Vitamins and herbal extracts can be added for their specific effects. Fragrance and therapeutic values are provided through the addition of pure essential oils. Very little essential oil is needed to make an aromatic water, and you can choose between citrus, herbaceous, floral, woodsy or balsamic aromas, or a blend of several.

Men in particular will appreciate the subtle aromas and refreshing feel of natural body splashes and tonics. Traditional herbs and spices such as bay, clove, nutmeg, lime, vanilla, pimento, cinnamon and sandalwood all lend their unique qualities to water- and alcohol-based splashes. You can choose to infuse only the herbs and spices, or to add essential oils for an extra dash of fragrance. Splashes also make great gifts for all occasions, and can be displayed in cut-glass brandy decanters and other decorative containers. They will keep their freshness and distinctive aroma for many years.

GENTLEMAN'S FAVORITE MORNING SPLASH

A brisk, refreshing morning splash. For all skin types.

- *4 oz. (120 ml.) witch hazel extract*
- *2 oz. (60 ml.) mineral water*
- *1/2 oz. (15 ml.) unflavored vodka*
- *1/2 oz. (15 ml.) vegetable glycerine*
- *10 drops bergamot PEO*
- *10 drops pimento berry PEO*
- *10 drops cinnamon PEO*
- *10 drops sandalwood PEO*
- *dried mixed spices (include your favorites: cinnamon sticks, vanilla beans, clove buds, allspice berries, nutmeg, star anise)*

Combine all ingredients in a measuring cup or beaker and stir well. Drop the dried spices into a decorative glass bottle, and pour the liquid over them. Use as needed.

BITTER ORANGE AND CLOVE AROMATIC TONIC

A fruity, aromatic tonic which can be used as a body splash, scalp tonic, skin refresher or eau-de-cologne. For all skin types. Use as desired.

- *6 oz. (180 ml.) witch hazel extract*
- *1 oz. (30 ml.) vegetable glycerin*
- *1 oz. (30 ml.) aloe vera gel*
- *20 drops clove bud PEO*
- *20 drops bitter orange PEO*
- *10 drops ylang-ylang PEO*

Mix all ingredients in a measuring cup and stir well. Pour into a glass bottle using a funnel, and cap. Shake the bottle before each use. Apply as needed.

LAVENDER BODY SPLASH

A fresh, clean all-over splash to use after a bath or shower.

- *4 oz. (120 ml.) witch hazel extract*
- *4 oz. (120 ml.) mineral water*
- *40 drops lavender PEO*
- *10 drops sandalwood PEO*

Combine all ingredients in a glass measuring cup or beaker, stirring well. Pour through a funnel into an 8 oz. glass bottle. Use the splash whenever you need a refreshing lift.

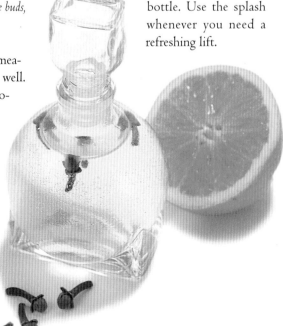

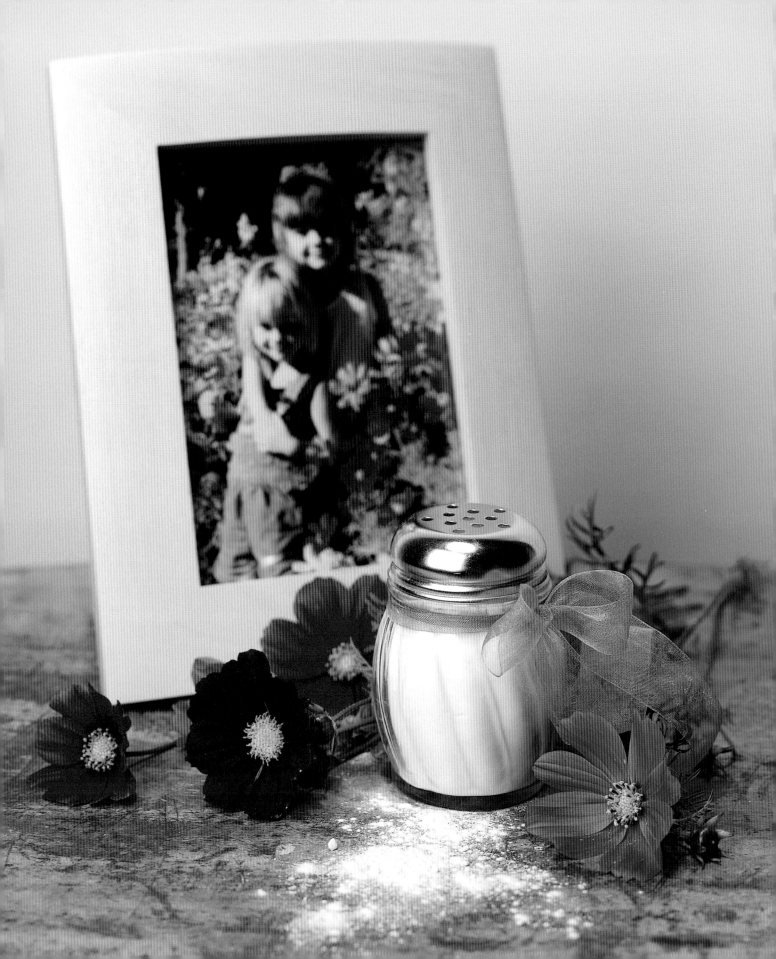

Dusting Powders

Men, women and children alike love the soft, luxurious feel of a silky dusting powder against clean skin. Body powders feel great after a bath or shower, or after sports and physical activities. Natural dusting powders are easy to make and have important advantages over similar products on the market. Commercial body powders often contain talc, a mineral that has been known to contain asbestos, a known carcinogen. Instead of taking risks with your health, make your own body powders using all-natural ingredients such as fine grain flours, starches and cleansing clays. An excellent base for a natural body powder is cornstarch and arrowroot powder, with white clay added. Rice starch and oat starch are pure, fine white powders which add elegance and 'hand feel' to powders. Fragrant essential oils add their clean botanical aromas and therapeutic advantages. Once made, display your powders in beautiful old-fashioned glass jars or antique salt shakers. If you are making powders for children's use, small salt and pepper shakers or plastic squeeze bottles are a good choice.

To make a natural body powder, combine the dry materials in a bowl, and blend together slowly using a metal whisk. Add the essential oils, taking care to count each drop. As you pour the drops into the mixture, stir them thoroughly into the powder to break them up and disperse them. Stir in concentric circles, bringing the powder from the edge of the bowl into the middle to ensure that all the powder is blended with the essential oils. Once the powder has acquired the desired fragrance strength, use a spoon to transfer it to your chosen decorative container. The powder will last months, and can be refreshed with essential oils at any time.

SPRINGTIME DUSTING POWDER FOR LINENS

A clean and fragrant powder for dusting upholstery, linens and pillows to make them smell like the first day of Spring!

- *1/2 cup (4 oz.) cornstarch*
- *1 Tbsp. white clay powder*
- *30 drops French lavender PEO*
- *30 drops rose geranium PEO*

Mix the ingredients together as described in Chapter Three ('Basic Dusting Powder'). Store in a glass shaker with perforated lid.

'FLOWER CHILDREN' GENTLE BODY POWDER

A soft, gently aromatic natural powder safe enough for children to use every day. Use in place of baby powder whenever a mild, absorbent powder is needed.

- *1/4 cup (2 oz.) cornstarch*
- *1/4 cup (2 oz.) arrowroot powder*
- *1 Tbsp. white clay*
- *30 drops sweet orange PEO*
- *20 drops ylang-ylang PEO*
- *10 drops rose geranium PEO*

Mix the dry materials together as described in the recipe above and stir in the essential oils. Use a clean, empty 'honey bear' plastic squeeze bottle or a pretty salt, pepper or cheese shaker bottle to store the powder.

ELEGANT ROSE PETAL DUSTING POWDER

An intensely fragrant powder for indulging your senses! Rice starch gives the powder a luxurious feel, and rose absolute its incredible uplifting aroma.

- *1/4 cup (2 oz.) cornstarch*
- *1/4 cup (2 oz.) rice starch*
- *20 drops rose geranium PEO*
- *12 drops rose absolute*

Mix the ingredients together, being sure to thoroughly blend in the rose absolute. Store this sensuous, fragrant body powder in an antique sugar shaker or old fashioned glass jar with a fluffy powder puff. Use the powder whenever you want to give your senses a real treat and make yourself feel truly special!

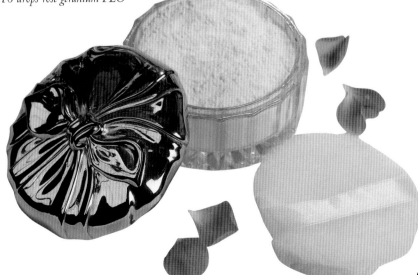

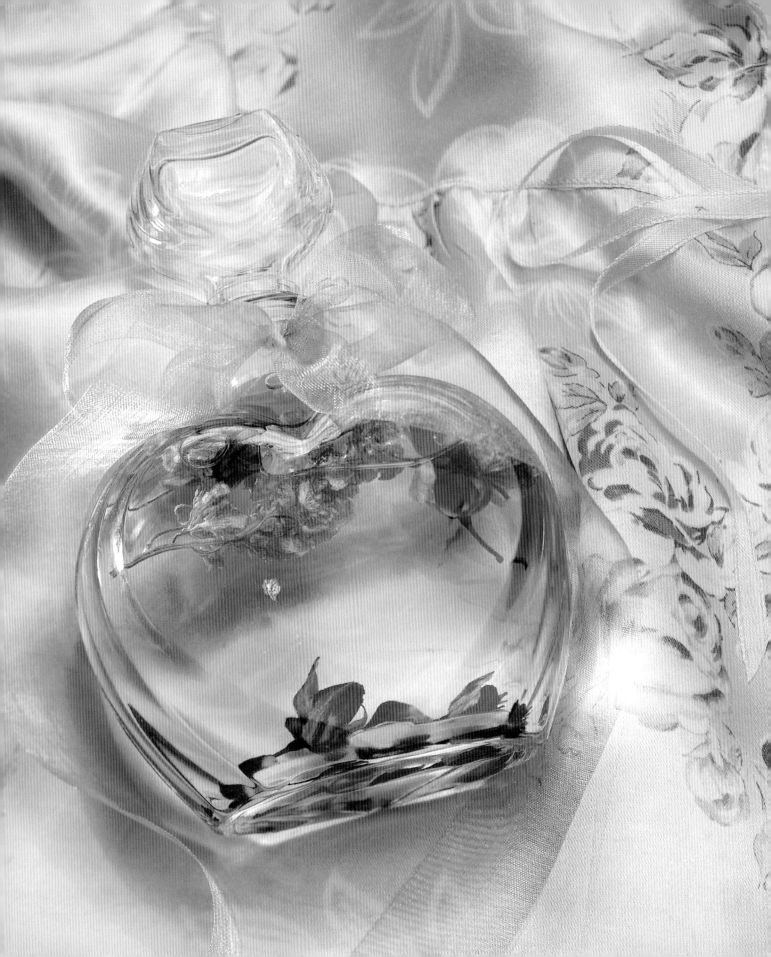

Body Oils

Most people are familiar with only two types of body oil — 'baby oil' and 'massage oil'. 'Baby oil' is mineral oil from petrochemical sources with a synthetic fragrance added. Mineral oil has been linked with acne and is also believed to leach vitamins from the body. While it has good qualities as a barrier oil to keep the skin from being affected by external elements, it is not a good choice as an allover body oil. Light, fine-textured oils from cold-pressed vegetable and nut sources are a much superior choice.

'Massage oils,' while mostly appropriate for their intended function, vary enormously in ingredient quality and overall effectiveness. While derived from natural sources, many massage oils are made with heat-treated or solvent-extracted oils that may also not be entirely fresh. Fatty acid peroxides (also known as 'free radicals') wreak major damage on oils that have been weakened by heat or chemical treatment, resulting in a shortened shelf life. You can easily recognize a peroxidized massage oil by its characteristic rancid smell, and in extreme cases, by the sticky, crystallized deposits between the neck of the bottle and the lid. Lengthy warehousing and transit times can also add to the deterioration of massage oil ingredients. While those with muscular aches and pains might appreciate the addition of warming substances like camphor and menthol to oils, too many commercial massage oils are fragranced with synthetic aromachemical fruit and flower scents, which are foreign to the body and are not recommended for application to permeable body skin. No heat- or chemical-treated oil, stale oil, or oil with synthetic fragrance additives should ever be used in the practice of professional full-body massage.

So how do you go about finding a first-class body oil for massage and skincare? Fortunately, the answer is simple. Nourishing body oils are incredibly easy to make yourself. Obtain the freshest cold-pressed vegetable, seed or nut oils you can find, add oil-soluble vitamins and special ingredients like phospholipids, herbal infused oils and pure essential oils and you will have created the ultimate body oil — in less than five minutes. Your body oil formula can be customized with the aromatherapeutic essences of your choice, and can be used for massage and general skincare, for scalp and hair treatments, hand and footcare, and as a bath oil.

DELUXE AROMATHERAPY MASSAGE OIL

A multipurpose oil designed to soothe and care for skin in need of nourishing treatment. Vitamin E and evening primrose oil add richness and texture. For all skin types.

- 6 oz. (180 ml.) *unfragranced body oil (see Chapter Three)*
- 1 oz. (30 ml.) *evening primrose oil*
- 1/2 tsp. *Vitamin E*
- 100 drops of the essential oils or blend of your choice

Mix all oils together in a beaker, stir and pour into a bottle. Apply liberally as needed.

SERENITY AROMATHERAPY SKINCARE OIL

This smooth, fine-textured oil has a fragrance reminiscent of orange orchards in full bloom!

- 8 oz. (240 ml.) *unfragranced body oil (see Chapter Three)*
- 30 drops *sweet orange PEO*
- 20 drops *East Indian sandalwood PEO*
- 20 drops *ylang-ylang PEO*
- 10 drops *neroli PEO*
- 10 drops *bitter orange PEO*
- 10 drops *vanilla oleo-resin*

Mix all the oils together, stir and decant into a glass bottle. This oil is an excellent oil to use after a bath or shower. A massage with 'Serenity' oil is a blissful, heavenly experience!

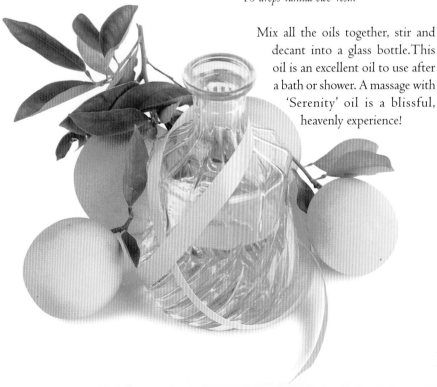

Lotions and Body Milks

Have you ever used a lotion frequently during the day, only to find that your skin actually feels increasingly dryer between applications? Your skin may not be the best candidate for commercial lotions containing mineral oil, synthetic scents and a variety of chemical ingredients in the formula. Sensitive skins in particular require a light natural lotion composed primarily of vegetable or nut oils, with a large complement of humectants and moisture factors. Dry skin types need a creamy lotion rich in cold-pressed oils with specialty oils and butters to nourish body skin with essential nutrients. Many people also prefer a lotion to an oil for bodycare. Vitamins and essential oils add anti-oxidant properties, therapeutic values and natural fragrance to lotion formulas.

Lotions for everyday use can be customized with a variety of essential oils to suit the needs of different skin types. Refer to the list on page 23 for recommendations of essential oils to blend into the unfragranced lotion base outlined in Chapter Three. Try your creativity making other types of lotions, such as body milks and perfumed voiles. Body milks are lighter, pourable lotions with a high water content. Perfumed voiles (or 'veils') are silky lotions with a higher concentration of natural fragrance, designed to be applied to the hands, arms and neck as a first 'layer' before applying perfume. The possibilities are endless — let your imagination be your guide!

FRENCH LAVENDER BODY MILK

Discreet and sophisticated, the fragrance of French lavender permeates this satiny lotion.

- *7 oz. (210 ml.) unfragranced body lotion (see Chapter Three)*
- *1 oz. (30 ml.) vegetable glycerin*
- *80 drops French lavender PEO*

Mix all ingredients together in a glass

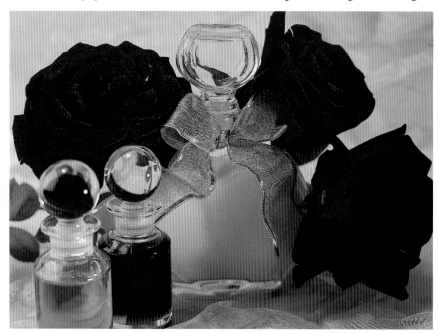

measuring cup or beaker. Stir well to blend. Pour the lotion into a glass bottle.

ORANGE BLOSSOM BODY LOTION

A silky body lotion with the soft, sensual fragrance of orange blossom. Sweet, warm and euphoric! For all skin types.

- *8 oz. (240 ml.) unfragranced body lotion (see Chapter Three)*
- *40 drops bitter orange PEO*
- *20 drops sweet orange PEO*
- *10 drops neroli PEO*
- *10 drops ylang-ylang PEO*

Mix all the ingredients together, pour into a glass bottle, and use as needed.

ROSE AND PATCHOULI SENSUOUS PERFUME VOILE

This sensual, exotic body lotion is made with rose, the Queen of Flowers, and blond Indonesian patchouli, known for its aphrodisiac qualities. Real Madagascar vanilla adds warmth, depth and vibrancy to the blend.

- *6 oz. (180 ml.) unfragranced body lotion (see Chapter Three)*
- *1 oz. (30 ml.) aloe vera gel*
- *1 oz. (30 ml.) vegetable glycerin*
- *20 drops vanilla oleoresin*
- *20 drops patchouli PEO*
- *20 drops rose geranium PEO*
- *8 drops rose absolute*

Mix all ingredients together in a glass measuring cup and stir with a whisk until well blended. The mixture should be liquid and silky. Pour the lotion into a decorative glass or crystal bottle. This exotic, aromatic beauty fluid is unsurpassed for fragrancing and softening the skin.

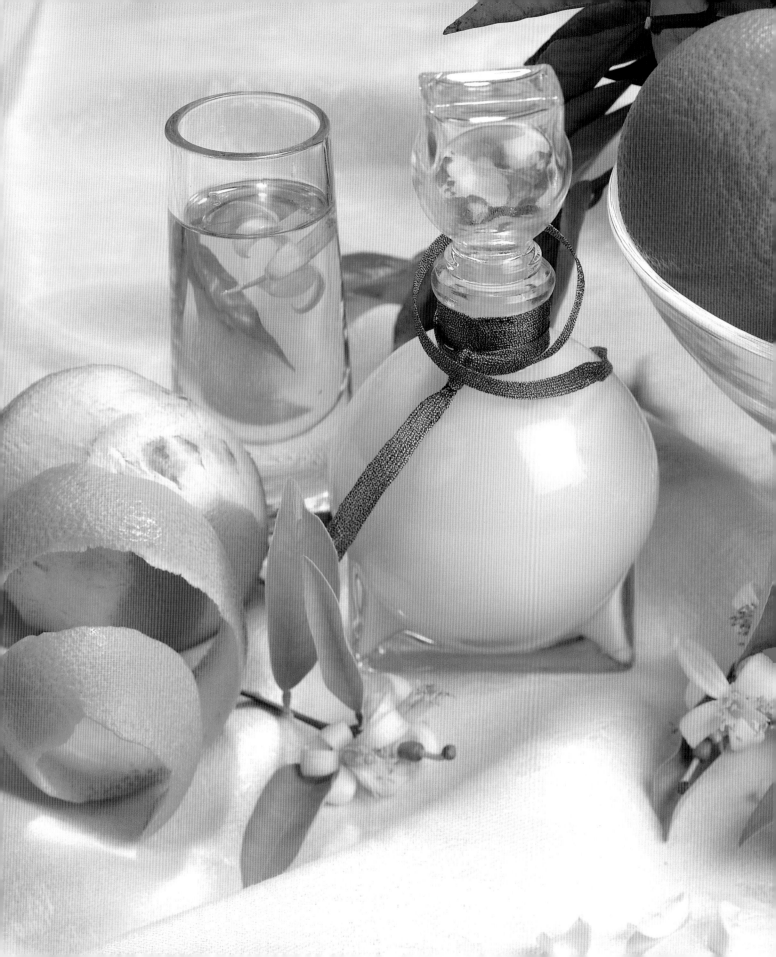

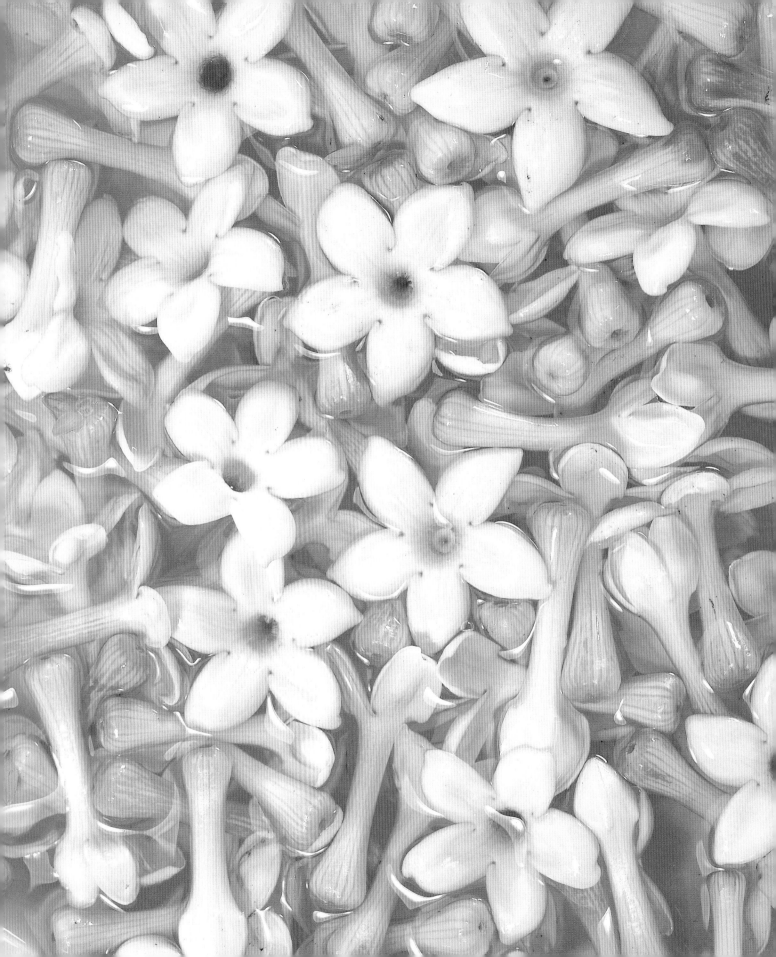

Infused Oils and Perfumes

Legend has it that Princess Nour Djihan, bride of the Mogul emperor Djihanguyr, noticed at her wedding that a shimmering film was forming over the palace pools where rose petals had been thrown. When skimmed from the water, the film held the incredible aroma of full-blown roses. 'Attar of roses,' as it became known, is a classic example of an infusion of flowers, in this case in water with warm sunshine accelerating the process. Infusion of flowers in oils and fats to make perfumes, unguents and ointments is one of the most ancient traditions. The Bible states that Mary Magdalen 'took a pound of ointment of spikenard, very costly, and anointed the feet of Jesus,' anointing with plant-infused ointments having the highest symbolism of respect and religious significance. During medieval times, medicinal herbs were routinely infused into unguents to use in the ongoing battle against plague and disease. One of the most popular plants for infusion is calendula, whose golden petals produce a healing, skin-regenerating oil. The famous 'Monoi' of Tahiti is made of coconut oil in which white gardenia blooms have been infused in the sun. Monoi is largely responsible for the radiant skin and luxuriant hair of the islanders. Enfleurage, the basis of much traditional perfume-making, employs the method of combining fragrant flowers with solid fats to extract their volatile aromas. These time-honored traditions are still practiced in countries around the world to this day.

You can try your hand at infusing flowers at home to create delicately fragrant infused oils. White flowers — gardenias, tuberose, stephanotis — are especially well suited to this technique. If you have a garden, experiment with old-fashioned roses and strongly-scented garden flowers and herbs. You can also make natural oil-based perfumes by combining this oil or a heavier oil such as jojoba with a few drops of precious absolutes such as rose, jasmine, orange blossom, carnation, hyacinth or narcissus. Solid perfumes can be made with the addition of melted beeswax. A drop or two of oakmoss, sandalwood, benzoin or vanilla will give your creations a wonderful depth and richness.

OIL OF WHITE FLOWERS

Pick unsprayed flowers early in the day, when their fragrance is at its peak, and place them in a shallow ceramic container with a clear glass lid. Pour golden olive oil over the flowers to cover them. Place the container in a warm place for one week. Using a wooden spoon, press the flowers to extract their essences, then strain them out of the oil and replace them with fresh ones. Repeat this procedure once or twice more. Once your oil has the gentle, characteristic aroma of the flowers, decant the oil through a funnel lined with cheesecloth into a glass bottle.

NATURAL PERFUME

You can customize the following recipe with any essential oil or exotic absolute or blend that you like.

- *1 oz. (30 ml.) refined jojoba oil*
- *20 drops absolute (or 50 drops essential oils, or blend)*

Pour the jojoba oil into a small bowl and pour in the drops of absolute or essential oil blend. Stir until thoroughly blended and decant into an attractive perfume decanter using a small funnel. You can also use unflavored vodka in place of the jojoba oil if you prefer an alcohol-based perfume. Rub drops on your wrists and pulse points as needed.

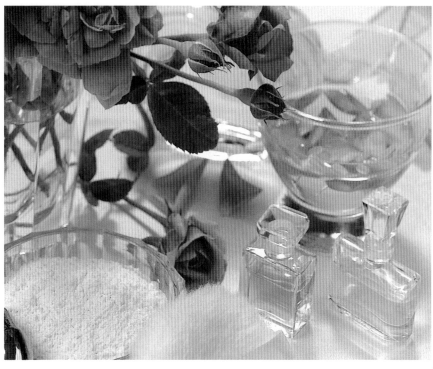

Chapter Seven
Hand & Footcare

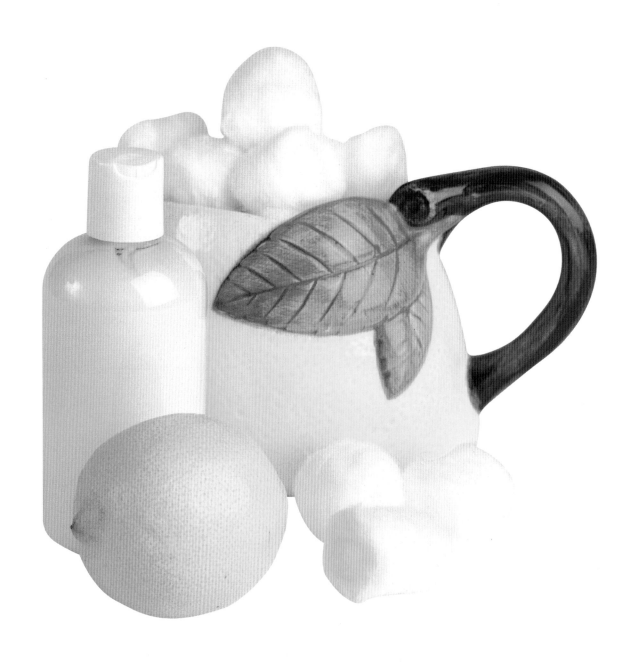

Introduction to Hand and Footcare

In today's stress-filled world, a visit to a salon for a professional manicure or pedicure is more than just a luxury — it provides a much-needed therapy, an opportunity to relax, unwind and be pampered while the world slips by outside. Have you ever wondered why a hand or foot treatment is so uniquely relaxing? Ever since humans became bipeds and started to use their hands to grasp, control and manipulate the world around them, our feet and hands have been doing extra duty! Rich in nerve endings, the hands are the outward extensions of our brain, endlessly moving, feeling and judging objects and situations. Our feet propel us forward through life as our eyes and mind take in the new horizons that surround us every step along the way. Actively involved in the flow of life, we choose to step heavily or lightly, to stumble or to dance. With life's hectic pace and the demands put on us daily, it's not surprising that we retreat as often as we can to the ancient ritual of just sitting, relaxing and allowing ourselves to be groomed and nurtured.

In the following pages, natural recipes are given for hand and foot cleansers, hydrotherapy baths, conditioning oils, lotions and aromatherapy treatments you can do at home. All the formulas use effective ingredients that naturally freshen, energize, moisturize and nourish the skin of arms, hands, legs and feet. Pure essential oils accomplish the task of destroying bacteria, disinfecting and deodorizing much better than many medicinal compounds on the market, and their fresh natural fragrances provide an added bonus. Water is the perfect carrier for the natural salts, herbs and oils used in the simple hydrotherapy treatments. Fresh, cold-pressed vegetable and nut oils, lecithin and oil-soluble vitamins strengthen the skin's ability to deal with the elements and renew itself properly. An ideal time for 'getting in touch' with your overworked hands and feet is the evening, when the TV is on and you are trying to put aside the stresses of the day in preparation for a new day tomorrow. You'll find that the recipes that follow will add to your sense of relaxation and renewal. Included here are basic reflexology charts for hand and foot massage. Reflexology, the study of improving well-being through stimulation of 'reflex points' on the feet, is a fascinating technique for dramatically improving your physical and mental health using simple and direct methods. Use the diagrams and recipes that follow for your own introduction to this healing art, and most of all, enjoy the experience!

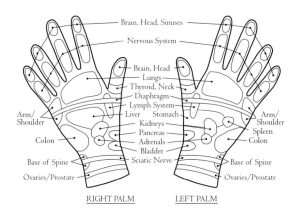

HAND REFLEXOLOGY CHART

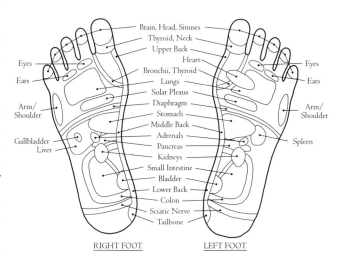

FOOT REFLEXOLOGY CHART

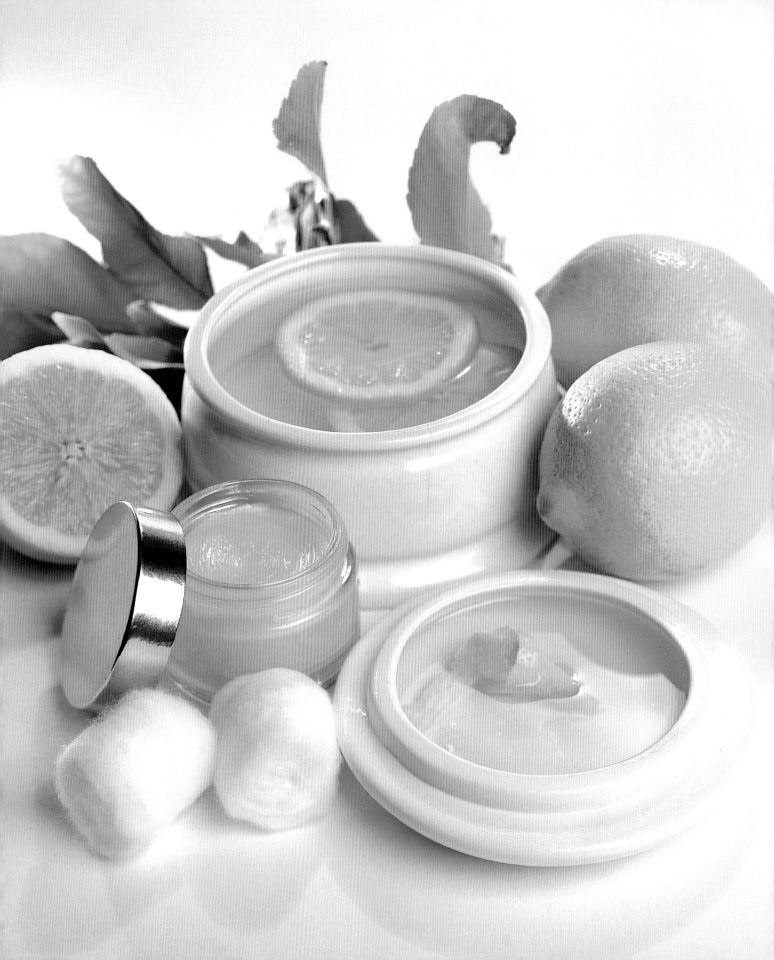

Nail Conditioning Treatments

Like the hair, nails are composed of keratin, a strong protein that is flexible and more resistant to the elements than the skin itself. Our translucent nails are a protective outgrowth of the fingertips, and they contain no nerves or live cells. The body of the nail is nourished by the nail bed on which it rests, and the underlying matrix, which contains nerve endings, blood and lymph. A healthy nail matrix will deliver vitamins, minerals and other nutrients to the nail bed. If the blood and lymph are rich in nutrients, and regular massage, care and maintenance are given to the hands and fingertips, the result will be smooth, strong, beautiful nails. Interestingly, the more the nails and surrounding cuticles are massaged and manipulated, the stronger and healthier the nails will become. Healthy, well-manicured nails provide an elegant finishing touch to our hands, which are constantly on display as we perform our daily tasks, assist others and express our thoughts and emotions.

Probably the plant most closely associated with hand and nail care is the lemon, and lemon juice is a key ingredient in most recipes dating back over the centuries. Lemon juice has anti-bacterial, deodorizing and bleaching qualities and is used to fade age spots, whiten skin and nails and stimulate healthy nail growth. Both lemons and the pure essential oil of lemon, expressed from the peel, are inexpensive and readily available.

SIMPLEST NAIL WHITENER

Cut a whole lemon in half, and press your fingernails into the cut half, rubbing cuticles and nails against the inner white portion of the peel. Massage your nails this way for several minutes before rinsing them under warm running water. Rough skin on elbows and knees can also be smoothed and softened by rubbing them with the cut lemon halves.

REFRESHING CITRUS NAIL SOAK

A fresh, anti-bacterial soak to deep-cleanse the skin and nails.

- *8 oz. (240 ml.) heated spring water*
- *juice of one lemon*
- *1 Tbsp. (15 ml.) aloe vera gel*
- *10 drops lemon PEO*

Mix the ingredients in a small container, and soak fingertips for 5 – 10 minutes.

LEMON OIL NAIL STRENGTHENER

A conditioning and strengthening warm oil treatment for healthy nails.

- *1/2 oz. (15 ml.) avocado oil, warmed*
- *1/2 tsp. Vitamin E*
- *10 drops lemon PEO*

Mix the carrier oils and lemon essential oil and pour into a small glass bottle with the cap on (but not tightly.) Stand the bottle in a half-full mug of just-boiled water. Pour the warmed oil into a small bowl and soak nails and fingertips for 5 – 10 minutes.

HEALING CITRUS NAIL AND HAND SALVE

A rich and nourishing 'barrier cream' for hard-working hands. Shea butter and lecithin give the salve its creamy, healing quality.

- *2 Tbsp. shea butter (or cocoa butter)*
- *1/2 oz. (15 ml.) hazelnut oil*
- *1/2 oz. (15 ml.) avocado oil*
- *1/2 tsp. modified lecithin*
- *30 drops lemon PEO*
- *30 drops mandarin PEO*

Melt the shea butter in a bain-marie and add the avocado and hazelnut oils. Stir in the lecithin, and when the mixture cools slightly, the lemon and mandarin essential oils. Store the salve in a wide-mouthed glass jar and apply as needed.

In addition to pure essential oil of lemon, have fun experimenting with other citrus oils:

- grapefruit
- bergamot
- mandarin
- lime
- sweet orange
- bitter orange
- blood orange

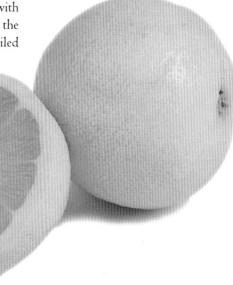

Hand and Foot Cleansers

Our hands and feet are frequently exposed to a great deal of strenuous activity, so it's wise to take special care of them, cleaning them thoroughly to remove dirt, grime and sweat, and softening them with water and cleansers to refine rough, chapped skin and to restore lost moisture. Like the rest of the body, skin on the hands and feet needs effective but gentle cleansing. The skin on the back of the hands is particularly thin and vulnerable and receives constant exposure to external elements, making hands the first part of the body to reveal aging. UV exposure, chemicals and detergents can also exact a harsh toll on the hands. Our feet are expected to support us through all our daily activities while encased in footwear that is sometimes constrictive and cumbersome. The result is often sweaty, aching feet that are susceptible to infections and irritations. The nerve endings in both feet and hands are particularly sensitive, so it's no wonder that a footbath or hand soak with softening cleansers feels so wonderful when we remember to treat ourselves to them!

Refreshing essences like peppermint, lemon, tea tree and rosemary are popular choices for hand and foot cleansers. The menthol content in peppermint provides a stimulating hot/cool sensation to weary, overworked feet. Here are a trio of recipes using pure essential oil of peppermint to deep-cleanse and refresh your deserving hands and feet.

GARDENERS' ROSEMARY AND PEPPERMINT CLEANSER

Green clay is an old-time favorite for absorbing dirt and soil on the skin and gently removing it. This liquid cleanser is a favorite of gardeners and anyone whose hands are exposed to oily dirt and grime.

- *8 oz. (240 ml.) unfragranced gel base (see Chapter Three)*
- *2 Tbsp. green clay powder*
- *25 drops rosemary PEO*
- *25 drops peppermint PEO*

Pour the gel base into a bowl and slowly stir in the clay powder and rosemary and peppermint oils until you reach a smooth consistency. Using a funnel, pour the mixture into a plastic squeeze bottle. Use in place of soap. Your skin will feel smoother, softer and cleaner overall.

PEPPERMINT AND BLACK WALNUT SCRUB

An invigorating scrub for feet and hands, with the brisk aroma of peppermint and the dirt-removing properties of black walnut hulls.

- *8 oz. (240 ml.) unfragranced gel base (see Chapter Three)*
- *3 Tbsp. black walnut hulls*
- *1 tsp. (5 ml.) modified lecithin*
- *50 drops peppermint*

Pour the gel base in a bowl and stir in the other ingredients until fully blended. Store the finished mixture in a wide-mouthed glass kitchen jar, and use a spoon to stir up the ingredients before using. Use with a washcloth or brush on the feet and on the palms of the hands as needed.

PEPPERMINT FOOT LOTION

This all-time favorite makes your tired feet feel like new! The addition of tea tree oil provides antibacterial benefits.

- *8 oz. (240 ml.) unfragranced lotion (see Chapter Three)*
- *1 tsp. (5 ml.) modified lecithin*
- *40 drops peppermint PEO*
- *20 drops tea tree PEO*
- *10 drops rosemary PEO*

Combine all ingredients in a measuring cup or beaker, stir well, and pour into a bottle. Use as needed to revive feet.

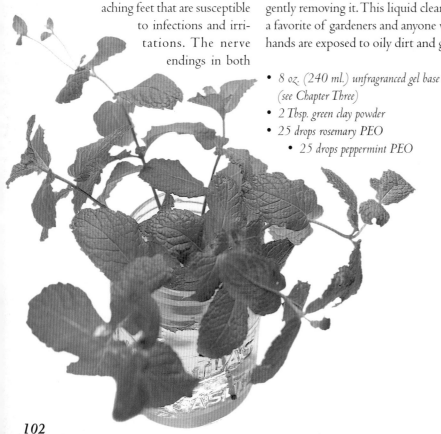

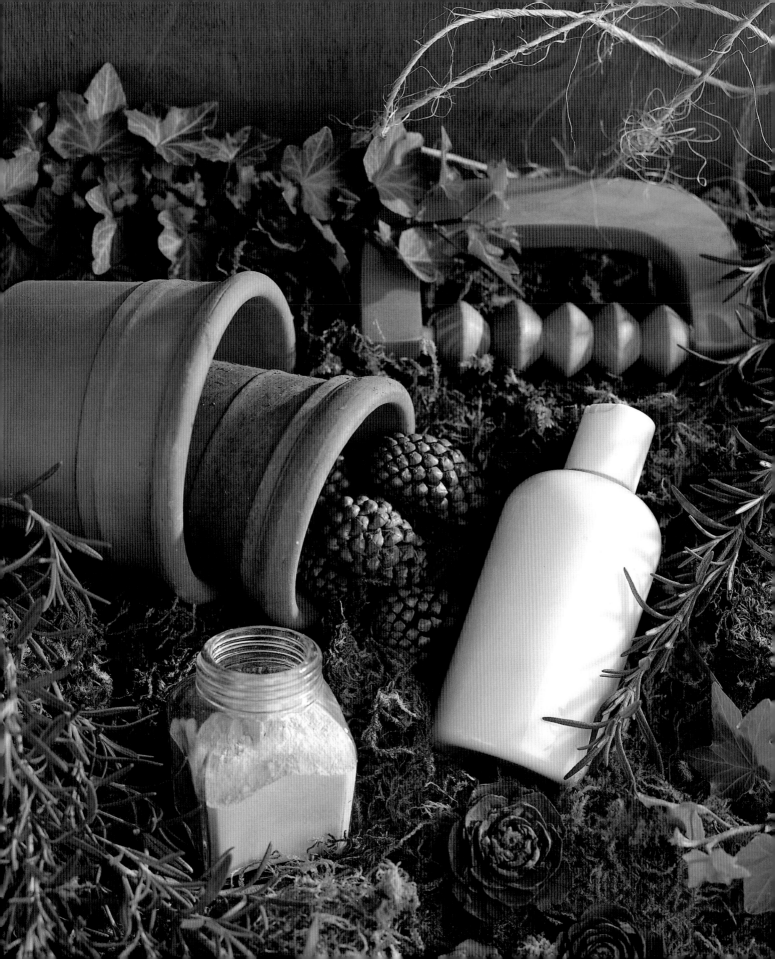

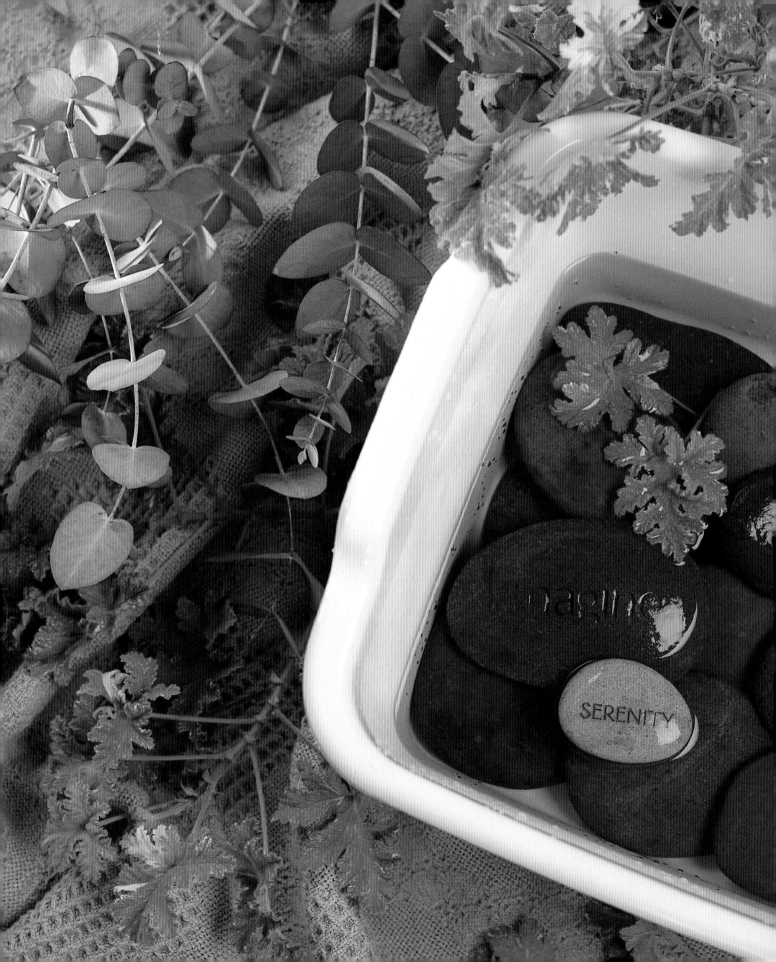

Hydrotherapy Hand and Foot Baths

While we take daily bathing and showering for granted, we tend to forget that our hard-working hands and feet are often in need of special therapeutic care. We use our hands constantly during the day, stretching, flexing and sometimes over-extending them through repetitive movements in the course of our work. Wrist and joint pain can result from overuse. We also underestimate the stress on our feet caused by long hours of standing, particularly in poorly-fitting shoes, or with bad posture. Feet in particular benefit greatly from customized footbaths containing healing substances such as mineral salts, natural sea salts, herbs and essential oils. Reflexology, the study and treatment of the hands and feet using massage of specific 'reflex points' is an excellent adjunct to home hydrotherapy footbaths. The central principle of reflexology is that all the organs of the human body can be energized, regulated and brought into balance through careful massage of the reflex points on the feet and hands. Next time you have had a particularly busy or stressful day, try an aromatherapeutic footbath and foot massage while you are unwinding and watching TV. Your feet will thank you!

MINERAL/HERBAL FOOTBATH
A therapeutic footbath with detoxifying mineral salts and purifying essential oils.

- *basin of hot water*
- *1/2 cup (4 oz.) coarse sea salts*
- *1/2 cup (4 oz.) Dead Sea mineral salts*
- *5 drops juniper berry PEO*
- *5 drops grapefruit PEO*
- *5 drops bitter orange PEO*

Stir the salts and oils into the basin of water and submerge your feet for 10 – 15 minutes. This combination of ingredients is detoxifying and may make you feel drowsy, so this is a good footbath to take before bedtime. Be sure to drink lots of water during and after the session. Finish with a foot massage with your choice of powder, oil or lotion.

AROMATIC REFLEXOLOGY FOOT SPA
A novel experience for overworked and aching feet. The heat of the water and the stones, and the therapeutic herb and flower oils combine to bring much-needed relief.

- *basin of hot water*
- *one dozen smooth stones, about 2" – 3" in diameter*
- *5 drops lavender PEO*
- *5 drops rosemary PEO*
- *3 drops lemongrass PEO*
- *3 drops geranium PEO*

Pour the hot water over the stones in a basin large enough to fit both feet comfortably, and stir in the essential oils. Submerge your feet, and once they start to feel relaxed, rotate your ankles, flex your toes and rub the insteps of both feet on the warmed stones. If you feel adventurous, you can give your feet an extra workout by trying to pick up the stones with your toes! After soaking feet, dry them off and treat them to a massage with powder, lotion or oil.

AROMATIC POT-POURRI HAND SOAK
This is a fragrant herbal 'tea' with bio-active elements to soothe and repair sensitive dry skin.

- *large bowl of warm water*
- *handful of mixed herbs to include rosebuds, lavender, marigold and chamomile*
- *3 drops lavender PEO*
- *3 drops chamomile PEO*
- *1 tsp. (5 ml.) infused calendula oil*

Place the herbs in a muslin drawstring bag, or add them directly to the water. Stir in the essential oils and infused calendula oil. Soak your hands up to the wrists in the mixture for 5 – 10 minutes. Rinse with warm water, towel dry and treat yourself to a hand massage with a nourishing lotion or cream. Your hands will feel relaxed and renewed.

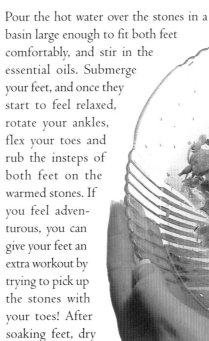
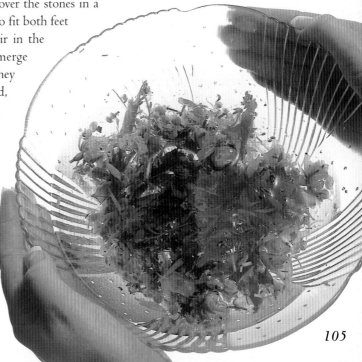

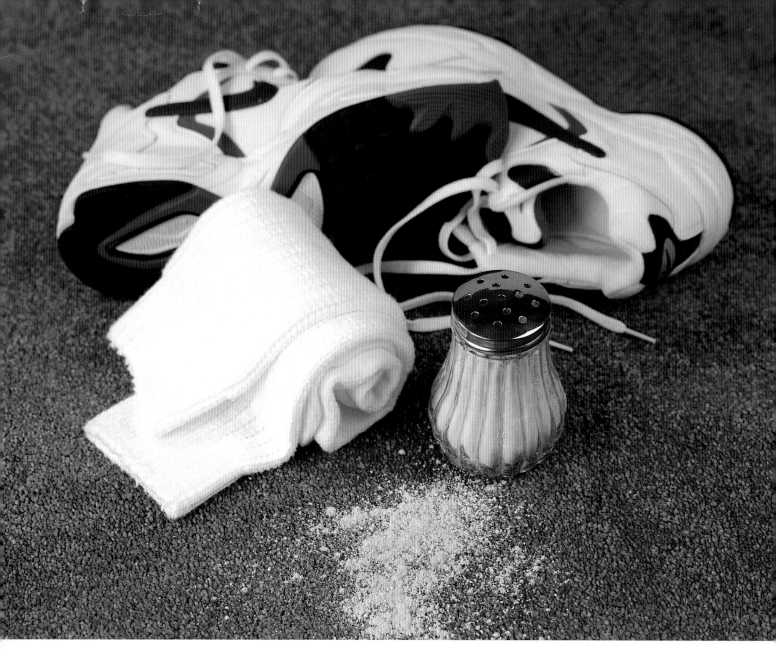

ESSENTIAL OILS FOR USE IN NATURAL FOOTCARE FORMULAS

For swelling and fluid retention:

- *juniper berry*
- *cypress*
- *lemon*
- *grapefruit*
- *petitgrain*
- *bitter orange*
- *chamomile*
- *rosemary*
- *yarrow*
- *valerian*

For itchy, infected skin:

- *tea tree*
- *rosemary*
- *lavender*
- *niaouli*
- *cajeput*
- *eucalyptus*
- *lemon*
- *marjoram*
- *thyme*
- *sage*

For sweaty, sticky skin:

- *peppermint*
- *spearmint*
- *sweet orange*
- *mandarin*
- *lemongrass*
- *sandalwood*
- *cedarwood*
- *lemon*
- *lavender*
- *geranium*

To fragrance and soften skin:

- *neroli*
- *lavender*
- *rose geranium*
- *sweet orange*
- *mandarin*
- *ylang-ylang*
- *sandalwood*
- *chamomile*
- *patchouli*
- *vanilla*

Foot Powders and Sprays

Foot problems are very common these days and stem from a variety of causes. One major and often-overlooked cause is the use of synthetic shoe materials which do not allow the feet to 'breathe' properly, resulting in damp and sweaty feet which provide a breeding ground for bacteria. Active and sports-oriented lifestyles mean that these problems are shared by more of the population than ever before. Fortunately, help is readily available in the form of pure essential oils — Nature's answer to infectious foot problems. The essential oils listed opposite can resolve a foot problem in a very short time and will keep your feet fresh, deodorized and resistant against the recurrence of athlete's foot and other skin conditions.

THERAPEUTIC FOOT POWDER

A medicinal powder that contains active elements to disinfect and heal inflamed and infected feet.

- *1/2 cup (4 oz.) arrowroot powder*
- *1 Tbsp. sea clay powder*
- *20 drops tea tree PEO*
- *10 drops white thyme PEO*
- *10 drops Spanish sage PEO*
- *10 drops lavender PEO*

Mix the powders in a bowl and whisk in the essential oils, drop by drop. Be sure to break up all the droplets of oil with the whisk. Once the powder is fully blended, spoon it into a wide-mouthed shaker jar (a cheese shaker works well) and cap tightly. Use as needed.

FRESH AND FRAGRANT FOOT POWDER

A silky floral-fragranced powder to use in the morning to keep feet cool and fresh all day long.

- *1/2 cup (4 oz.) cornstarch*
- *1/2 cup (4 oz.) rice starch*
- *1 Tbsp. white clay powder*
- *20 drops ylang-ylang PEO*
- *20 drops mandarin PEO*
- *10 drops neroli PEO*

Mix the powders in a bowl and whisk in the essential oils, drop by drop. Rotate the whisk slowly around the bowl in concentric circles to break up the oil droplets and blend them well into the powders. Once all the ingredients are completely blended, spoon into a shaker jar and cap tightly. This powder is excellent to use in the morning before putting on your shoes. It also makes a fragrant and long-lasting powder for scenting linens and upholstery, and can be sprinkled on tissues and tucked into closet drawers for freshness.

CITRUS ALOE SPRAY

A refreshing, deodorizing spray for sweaty, sticky hands or feet.

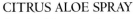

- *7 oz. (210 ml.) distilled water*
- *1 oz. (30 ml. aloe vera gel*
- *60 drops mandarin PEO*

Combine all ingredients and pour through a funnel into an 8 oz. plastic bottle. Spray on as needed.

EUROPEAN FRICTION RUB AND SPRAY

Many people suffer from swelling of hands, feet and ankles as a result of circulatory problems, weather fluctuations and long-distance air travel. Essential oils, herbal extracts and alcohol create a 'friction rub' which reduces fluid retention and inflammation.

- *4 oz. (120 ml.) distilled or spring water*
- *1 oz. (30 ml.) witch hazel extract*
- *1 oz. (30 ml.) aloe vera gel*
- *1 oz. (30 ml.) unflavored 90-proof vodka*
- *1 tsp. (5 ml.) polysorbate 20*
- *20 drops juniper berry PEO*
- *20 drops lavender PEO*
- *20 drops chamomile PEO*
- *20 drops grapefruit PEO*

Pour all liquids into a glass measuring cup and whisk until blended. Use a funnel to decant the mixture into a bottle. Shake well before each use. To use, splash the liquid into the palms of both hands and briskly massage the swollen areas for several minutes until the swelling subsides. To convert the rub into a spray, attach a spray mister to the bottle and spray the affected areas. The liquid evaporates from the skin, leaving a cool, fresh feeling.

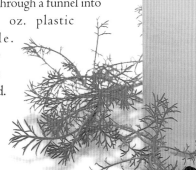

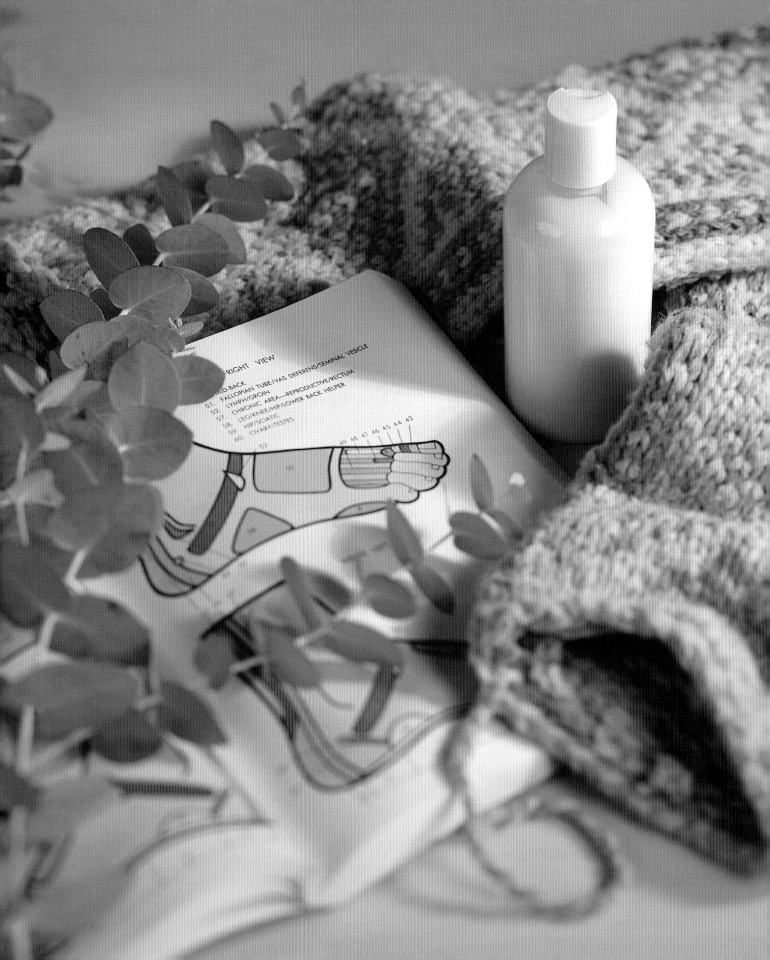

Hand and Foot Lotions

Our hands are one part of our bodies that are almost constantly exposed — to water, household chemicals, and external elements like wind, sun and pollution. Unless we moisturize and protect them, they very quickly show signs of premature aging. You can check the condition of your skin by pinching a fold of skin on the back of your hand and seeing how quickly the skin returns to normal. If it takes awhile, consider supplementing your diet with Vitamins C and B complex and applying a rich hand lotion daily until you see improvement. If your occupation exposes your hands to a great deal of repetitive, active or outdoor work, be sure to use a rich hand lotion or barrier cream frequently. If you want to add an SPF (Sun Protection Factor) to hand creams, an effective addition to formulations is p-methoxycinnamate, a natural substance derived from cinnamon. Each 1% of p-methoxycinnamate added to your base lotion will increase its SPF by two. A recipe for a nourishing hand cream with an SPF factor of 8 is given below.

We often overlook our feet, but they can benefit from a massage using a penetrating aromatherapy lotion. When you first begin to massage your feet, you may be surprised at how many sensitive spots you find, particularly on the soles of your feet and around the heels and ankles. If you are not familiar with reflexology (the study of correcting imbalances in the body through massage of special points on the feet and hands,) several excellent reflexology books may be found in your local book store. A basic knowledge of reflexology will greatly enhance your hand and foot massages. Adding essential oils to your lotions and creams is also important, as the essential oils are absorbed directly in the areas you are massaging, providing aromatherapeutic benefits as well. After massaging your feet until the lotion is completely absorbed, keep them warm by putting on a pair of socks or slippers and relaxing with your feet up.

HAND LOTION WITH SPF 8
Ideal protection for your hands! This formula contains rich moisturizers, antioxidant vitamins, and a natural sunscreen.

- *8 oz. (240 ml.) unfragranced body lotion (see Chapter Three)*
- *2 tsp. p-methoxycinnamate*
- *1/2 tsp. modified lecithin*
- *1/2 tsp. Vitamin A*
- *1/2 tsp. Vitamin E*
- *50 drops sandalwood PEO*
- *30 drops rosewood PEO*
- *20 drops lavender PEO*

Pour the unfragranced lotion into a bowl and stir in the lecithin, vitamins and the p-methoxycinnamate. Then add the essential oils drop by drop, stirring constantly. When the mixture is fully blended, pour it through a funnel into a bottle and cap tightly. Use as needed.

HERBAL REFLEXOLOGY LOTION FOR FEET AND HANDS
This fresh, clean-smelling lotion contains nourishing ingredients to treat your feet and hands, as well as pure essential oils to stimulate and energize.

- *8 oz. (240 ml.) unfragranced body lotion (see Chapter Three)*
- *1 oz. (30 ml.) aloe vera gel*
- *1/2 tsp. modified lecithin*
- *50 drops eucalyptus PEO*
- *25 drops lemon PEO*
- *20 drops tea tree PEO*
- *15 drops peppermint PEO*
- *10 drops rosemary PEO*

Pour the unfragranced lotion, aloe vera gel and lecithin into a bowl, and add the essential oils, drop by drop. Stir well until the lotion is completely blended. Pour through a funnel into a bottle and cap tightly. Apply as needed. When massaging feet and hands, use deep, small circular motions, and apply gentle but firm pressure to sore points. Continue until the lotion has been fully absorbed. Finish your massage with long, sweeping strokes away from the body.

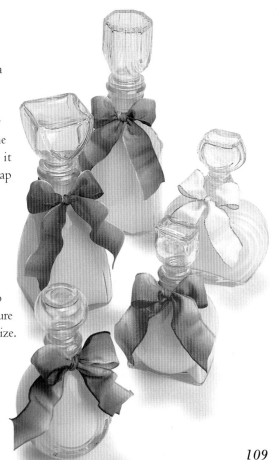

Chapter Eight

Creating Natural Bodycare Gifts

Once you have experimented with several of the recipes in this book and created some custom bodycare formulas of your own, you'll naturally want to share them with your family and friends. A large part of the fun of learning how to make bath and body products lies in designing your own recipes to make for special occasions, and creating the whole package, from the product ingredients and containers right through to your personalized gift presentation. With a little preparation and imagination, you can put together a stunning gift basket yourself, and for much less money than a commercial gift basket would cost. Not only will you save money, but your personalized gifts are sure to be appreciated more than most mass-produced items, will be used often and will create warm memories that will be treasured for years to come. There's something special about a gift that has been exclusively designed for someone by a friend or relative who knows them well and has created a heartfelt gift, especially one that will have a positive impact on their health and well-being.

When you start to make gifts of your natural bodycare creations, your perception of packaging and containers will be radically altered! You'll begin to see new uses for all types of containers that you might have at home or in the garage. Yard sales and flea markets will be overflowing with useful packaging ideas; you'll even notice the diversity of shapes and styles of bottles and jars at your local grocery. Antique stores, cooking and gardening shops and specialty stores will give you ideas for one-of-a-kind gift materials and packaging. Thrift stores, import gift emporiums and discount stores always carry a wide array of affordable and unique containers, including woven baskets, pots and tins. Fabrics, ribbon, decorative trim, labels and markers are all inexpensively found at local fabric and crafts stores, stationers and office suppliers. Outdoor nurseries, builders supply and hardware stores and florists can provide natural materials, unusual containers and a wide array of fresh and dried botanicals. Best of all, many natural decorative elements are waiting to be discovered outdoors, in the garden, in the woods or at the seashore. You are the chemist, creator and manufacturer — let your gifts be a true expression of your personal style!

You may choose to personalize your gift baskets to a particular theme, a holiday or special occasion, to meet a health or beauty need or simply to let someone know that you care and are thinking of them. Your natural bodycare gifts will be all the more appreciated if all your creations are attractively labeled with a descriptive name and ingredient disclosure. It's a nice touch to include the date you made the products, and maybe some additional information about interesting ingredients or the aromatherapy effects of your formulas. Ingredient disclosures list all the ingredients in the product, starting with the ingredient having the largest percentage present in the formula, and continuing until you have listed all ingredients by quantity in descending order. For good visual effect, handwrite your instructions using waterproof permanent ink on sticky labels or tie-on tags. Don't forget to add 'patch test' instructions for sensitive individuals, if you suspect that they might be allergic to any substance. To perform a patch test, simply rub a small amount of the product on the inside of the elbow or wrist, cover with a small adhesive bandage, and wait 24 hours. If redness or skin irritation occurs, do not use.

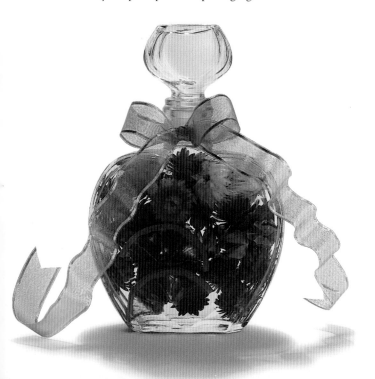

Reasons for giving your natural gifts are as numerous as days in the year, and can range from small thoughtful sentiments, such as showing appreciation to a new employee or cheering a housebound neighbor, through to grander statements appropriate for a much-awaited family reunion, anniversary or special achievement. Your custom-designed gifts are sure to be welcome on birthdays, at Christmas, Thanksgiving, Mother's Day, Father's Day, Valentine's Day and many other holiday occasions. Along with the seasons, we all celebrate the many stages of our lives — birth, religious events, high school and university graduation, marriage, housewarming, job promotion, children, hospital stays, illnesses, moving, retirement — even our passing. You can bring a special meaningfulness to life's events, large or small, by creating your own personalized natural bodycare gifts, displayed with verve and originality and given with caring and joy. Everybody's creative awareness and manner of expressing their design talents is different, so this book provides some visual examples of gift baskets as well as a series of design 'checklists' to assist you in selecting your packaging components and inspiring you to create new and different looks for each gift.

Once you have decided on a gift for a special occasion, give some thought to the recipients' tastes and desires. What are your friends' lifestyles and occupations? Do they have stressful jobs, or do they travel or commute a lot? How old are they, are they single or married, free-spirited or family-oriented, and do they live in the city or country? What are their likes and dislikes? What hobbies do they have, and are they the stay-at-home indoors types or active outdoors nature lovers? Do they like to pamper themselves with spa treatments, or are they rugged individualists who are only familiar with bar soap? What types of aromas do you think they might appreciate — floral, fruity, herbaceous, spicy, woodsy or exotic? With this information as a basis, you can start to put together ideas for natural bodycare products they'll enjoy, with a theme to tie everything together. Here are some ideas:

Gardener's pot of goodies: An ideal gift for a man or woman who loves to garden and be outdoors, a glazed green flowerpot holds bottles of homemade shower gel and lotion made with clean-smelling essential oils of herbs and flowers. Use sphagnum moss, shredded wood fibre or excelsior as a base for your display. Tuck a flax or cotton washcloth and terra-cotta foot scrubber into the pot, together a couple of simple related items such as a wooden comb and a green clay soap with a nature motif. For added emphasis, decorate your gift pot with sprigs of eucalyptus, ivy, rosemary or evergreens such as cypress, pine or fir. Other additions, depending on the size of the

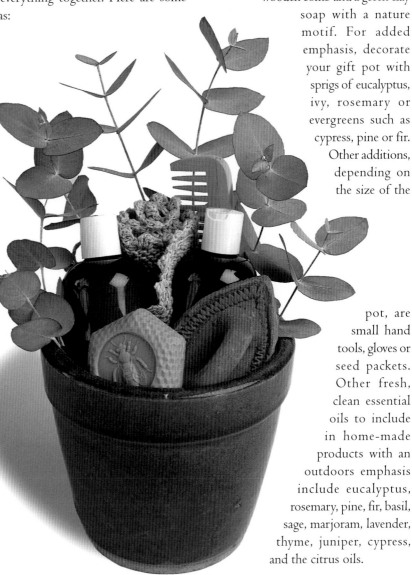

pot, are small hand tools, gloves or seed packets. Other fresh, clean essential oils to include in home-made products with an outdoors emphasis include eucalyptus, rosemary, pine, fir, basil, sage, marjoram, lavender, thyme, juniper, cypress, and the citrus oils.

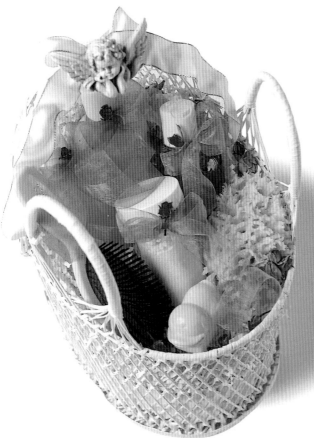

Gift bassinet for a baby shower:

Natural bodycare products are ideal for babies and make a thoughtful and caring customized gift. Dusting powder, natural skincare oil, lotion and ultra-mild bathing gel are packaged in unbreakable clear plastic bottles and decorated with gauzy pastel ribbon. Use mild, soft, floral oils in these recipes — lavender, chamomile or orange blossom, for example. Include a soft natural sea sponge, hairbrush or whimsical animal nailbrush. A small illustrated book, booties, embroidered washcloth or rattle make nice additions if you have a larger container. Search crafts and floral supply stores for unusual basket shapes like this light wicker bassinet, then decorate it with tassels, ribbon, or a little guardian angel, display your gifts on soft cloud-like cotton or shredded paper, and finish with a little sprinkling of soft pink rosebuds!

Market basket for a city dweller:

A wicker basket sets the mood for someone who loves the country and wishes he or she could spend a day at a farmer's market rather than a corporate board meeting! Fresh citrus products will revive a disillusioned city dweller. A natural wicker basket contains an array of body products containing pure essential oil of sweet orange. A large decanter of massage oil filled with decorative dried orange slices and flowers backs up bottles of homemade orange-scented lotion, gel and room spray. A round orange soap ball wrapped in rust-colored fabric, small orange bedside candle, crisp cream tissue and slices of preserved orange fruit complete the presentation.

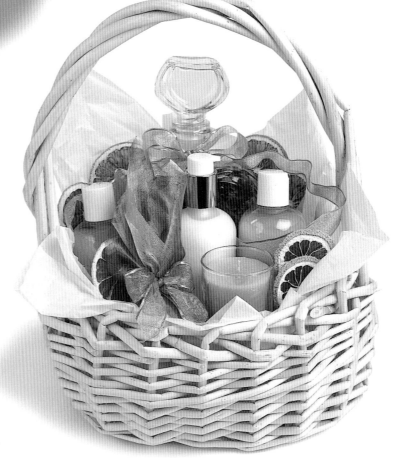

Anti-stress basket for the executive: Reward a hard worker with a metal tray basket filled with sybaritic products to relieve all that job stress! Select a soothing aromatherapy essential oil — lavender for example — and use it as the focus for your theme basket. Include a bottle of lavender massage and skincare oil, a refreshing room spray, lotion for dehydrated skin and dusting powder for sweaty feet. Improve office air quality with a bouquet of dried lavender or small sachet bag to keep on the desk, and a lightbulb ring with essential oil of lavender to use with a table lamp. A lavender silk eye pillow, wooden back massager and tape of ambient or classical music are welcome additions to quiet 'time out' breaks from the everyday routine. The metal tray basket is recyclable — you'll probably need to fill it up again the same time next year!

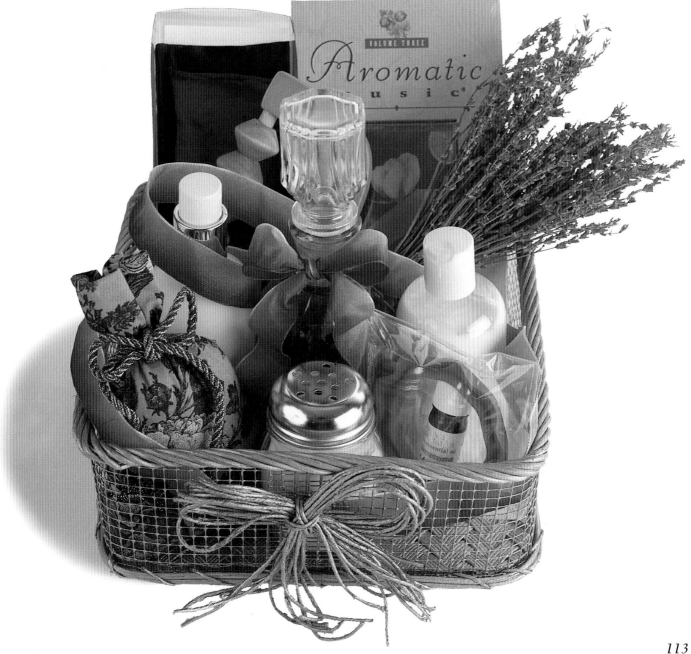

Here are some ideas for unusual containers in which to package your custom oils, perfumes, body lotions, bath salts and powders:

- bottles and jars; old, new and recycled
- antique apothecary jars and pharmacy bottles
- ceramic and porcelain pots with lids
- perfume atomizers, boudoir bottles, inkwells
- decorative tea cups, saucers, bowls and dishes
- cut-glass brandy decanters and liquor bottles
- old-fashioned kitchen containers, jugs and pitchers
- spice shakers, salt and pepper shakers
- mason jars, jam and jelly jars
- cake and biscuit tins, tobacco tins
- large seashells

Once you have made and packaged your products, you'll want to display them in a larger, sturdy container suitable for gift-giving. Keep an eye open for the following to add to your collection:

- woven baskets of all kinds; natural or painted
- terra-cotta flowerpots and saucers
- ceramic bowls and vases
- wooden and metal boxes and crates
- hat boxes and tote bags
- florist's buckets and ice buckets

Packing materials run the gamut from earthy and natural to crisp and sophisticated. Try these for different visual effects:

- shredded wood fibre, 'excelsior,' wood chips, moss
- corrugated cardboard strips, shredded paper or tissue
- dried potpourri, leaves, grasses and flowers
- cotton batting, burlap, muslin and gauze
- colored tissue, metallic tissues and papers
- clear, colored or printed cellophane sheets

Finishing your products and containers with natural fabrics always gives a polished, professional look. There are numerous textures of fabrics to choose from:

- natural fabrics: unbleached cotton, muslin, linen
- deluxe fabrics: silks, velvets, embroidered fabric
- delicate fabrics: lace, voile, gauze, netting, metallics
- 'theme' fabrics: printed cottons and gingham

Similarly, ribbons and ties provide a rich finishing touch to your products and theme baskets. Select from a wide range of aesthetic looks:

- raffia, string or jute; natural or colored
- satinized or metallic cord or braid
- narrow 'hair ribbon' in many colors
- French-wired ombré and luxury ribbons
- mini-pearl rope, beaded cord, tassels

Decorative elements often provide the final flourish which gives a gift its unique character and charm. Keep a collection of little 'found objects' that you can tie on as a distinctive memento:

- dried or silk flowers, twigs, berries, spice sticks
- seedpods, nuts, cones, feathers, birds' eggs
- stones, crystals, seashells, beads, coins, tokens
- miniature craft items, toys, keys, fetishes
- Oriental spoons and wooden scoops

Labeling your products is important and can be accomplished with style! Here are some ideas for unique, attractive label materials and lettering techniques:

- antique reproduction labels with decorative borders
- photocopies of antique designs (from your local library)
- decoupaged magazine clippings on sticky labels
- custom rubber-stamped labels in different colors
- gold or silver foil and aluminum garden plant tags
- tie-on 'necklace' labels made of different materials
- handmade floral, marbled and Oriental papers
- metallic ink messages on kraft or natural papers
- old-fashioned calligraphic script in colored ink
- writing directly onto bottles with indelible ink

Last but not least, you may want to select a theme that meets the individual interests of the person who'll be receiving your gift. Listed below are a variety of subjects which may provide inspiration:

- Nature: the outdoors, gardens, trees, flowers, herbs
- animals: cats, dogs, farm animals, birds
- symbols: geometric shapes and motifs, hearts
- natural elements: seasons, sun, moon, stars
- colors: metallics, brights and pastels
- travel, fashion, glamour, accessories
- history, special events, holidays, reunions
- tropical themes, spas, vacations, leisure
- hobbies and personal interests

Bear in mind that often, the simplest, most unique ways of creating gifts of your bodycare products are often the most memorable. For example, you may have created a fragrant aromatherapy massage oil for a friend, which, while it smells wonderful, looks a little bland in a plain plastic bottle. Why not give it a special cachet by pouring it into a new or recycled decorative glass bottle instead? The bottle can then be 'dressed up' with a ribbon bow, gold cord, decorative label, or little bunch of flowers or herbs tied around its neck. Another fun technique is to select naturally colorful dried flowers and herbs (they must be completely dry to avoid spoiling the oil), arranging them inside the gift bottle using a chopstick. After you've completed your dried flower display, gently tip the bottle to remove any small broken pieces of flowers or leaves, then slowly pour the massage oil into the bottle using a funnel. Once the bottle is

full, leave it for a few minutes for air bubbles to rise, refill if necessary, then wipe the top clean and cap or cork your bottle. This technique also works well using seashells, marbles, or any other dry, non-porous items. Once you have completed your gift, be sure to label or tag it, and finish it off with a luxurious ribbon bow.

The beauty of this presentation is that your healthy and useful gift makes a spectacular display in the bathroom or bedroom, and can be easily refilled with more aromatherapy oil as needed.

Whether as simple as a bottle of bodycare oil or as elaborate as a theme basket filled with an array of your products, the energy, inspiration and creativity you will bring to your gift designs are sure to be appreciated and remembered for years by all the lucky people who receive them!

Chapter Nine
Living the Natural Lifestyle

Now that you have tried and tested some of your own recipes and received positive feedback from friends and family who've used them as well, you'll have become aware that natural bodycare is not just a fad or gimmick — it is a integral and rewarding part of a healthy, holistic way of life. Making your own natural bodycare products is more than just a satisfying pastime; it has creative, therapeutic and health-promoting effects as well. Once you see the positive effects your own body-care products have on your appearance and well-being, you will probably want to learn more about other ways you can begin to shift your thinking and start to live your life in a manner that is more in tune with the natural world. Whether you are a city dweller or an urban refugee, there are numerous ways you can practically and realistically get back in touch with nature. All of these changes are within reach and can be accomplished easily and painlessly. In addition, you'll know that the changes you make are going to have positive lasting effects on your health, quite possibly even extending your life many years.

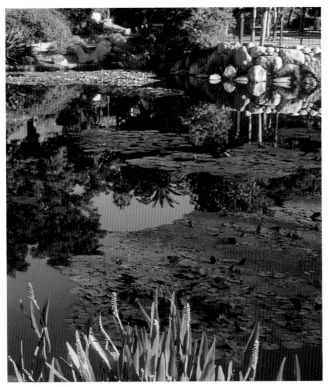

LEARNING TO LIVE THE NATURAL LIFE

Most of us in the western world are caught up in a fast-paced, urgent way of life. We rush from place to place, not taking the time to think, eat, breathe or relax properly. Everything is accomplished on the run as we race through our daily checklist of activities. Our jobs are stressful, our working environments often unhealthy or unharmonious, and we feel as if something is missing despite the energy we put into being productive. There never seems to be enough time to spend with the family, and when we do have the time, we may feel guilty, exhausted or unable to enjoy ourselves. We can feel overburdened by financial, relationship and health pressures, and see no way out of any number of difficult situations, real or imagined. The problem with this way of life is that we have fallen seriously out of touch with ourselves, our needs and our core being. The pressure of living life this way takes its toll on our physical, mental and emotional health and prevents us from getting in touch with ourselves and our real reasons for being alive on the planet.

The promises of science and technology have been fulfilled in many ways, and we have definitely benefited from their many contributions to our lives. Regardless, we still have less leisure time than ever before, and our stress levels have never been higher. The medical profession now acknowledges that stress is the number one cause of illness in our society. The past few years have seen the development of numerous ways to manage stress and create health and harmony in every aspect of our lives. For increasing numbers of people, these ways center on a renewed appreciation of the natural world — its simplicity, lack of pretense, truth and myriad means of self-expression. Many people are seeking a renewed sense of balance through natural diet, movement and exercise, alternative therapies, meditation, holistic stress management techniques, and many other ways of realizing full physical, mental, emotional and spiritual health. After many years of scientific and technological progress, as we enter the new millenium, we are now opening to a realm of the senses, allowing ourselves to integrate our lives with the positive aspects of the natural world in order to realize balance, healing and well-being.

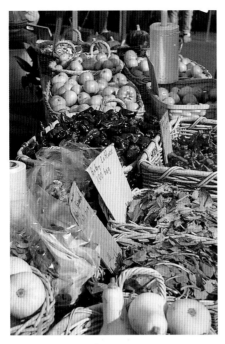

DIET AND NUTRITION

If a life-long pattern of holistic health begins with avoidance of unnecessary chemicals in our personal care products, household goods and fragrances, it only makes sense to avoid them in the foods we put into our bodies as well. Modern 'convenience' foods, which often lack any nutritive value, contain refined sugars or excess salt, hydrogenated fats, synthetic flavors and colors and many other chemical additives that are detrimental to our health. Pesticides and other 'agri-chemicals' are present in an alarmingly high percentage of the foods we buy, while valuable vitamins, minerals and nutrients are lost or destroyed in food processing. Deep-frying also damages foods' nutritive value. Many chemicals used in the food and beverage industry are not well accepted by the body, resulting in the build-up of toxins and waste materials in the body tissues. This creates a vicious cycle where we feel constantly 'under par',

fatigued and lethargic, unable to summon the energy to eat right, exercise, get out in the world and enjoy life.

To correct this situation, make a point to consciously think about all the food you purchase and consume every day. In many industrialized countries, over-eating or eating the wrong foods has become a preoccupation and pastime, satisfying needs beyond basic sustenance, to the great detriment of our general health. Try as much as possible to buy fresh foods that are in their naturally-occurring states, and plan meals accordingly. Emphasize high-quality proteins, whether of animal or vegetable origin, as well as simple carbohydrates and fresh fruits and vegetables. Be sure to drink plenty of pure water in addition to fresh juices and herb teas, keeping alcohol, coffee and soft drinks to a minimum. Re-educate your taste buds and avoid fast, fried and junk foods in favor of healthy alternatives. Health food

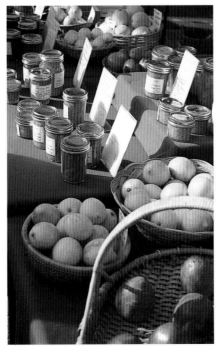

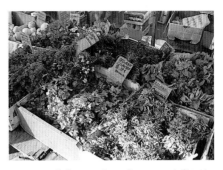

stores and farmers' markets specialize in organic and fresh-grown produce. Your body/mind needs the best fuel available to ensure its continued good health!

Since our bodies and minds do not function optimally without good nutrition, it is critical to know your own unique nutritional needs to compensate for any deficiencies and to allow nutritive food supplements to assist in your preventive health program. If you have a pre-disposed, genetic or medical condition which would benefit from special supplementation, make it your business to research it yourself or with the assistance of a responsive professional, so that you can identify the supplements you need. Herbs, vitamins, minerals, amino acids and a wide range of exciting new 'nutraceutical' and 'anti-aging' compounds can offer you definite physical and mental health advantages. Most of these substances (e.g., ginseng, echinacea, fever-few, ginkgo biloba, St. John's Wort, to name a few) are derived from natural sources and potentized with the help of modern technology, offering us the best of both worlds. So, whether you are growing herbs in pots or a windowbox to add to home-cooked meals, or whether you have a sophisticated 'internal body-care' supplement program, you are doing your health a favor and are taking the holistic route to natural wellness.

EXERCISE AND MOVEMENT

Regular exercise goes hand in hand with good diet and nutrition and is integral to achieving and maintaining good health. Lack of exercise contributes to, and sometimes causes, a host of health-destroying ailments. Proper exercise on the other hand, offers a multitude of health benefits. It conditions and tones the body, burns calories, improves the health of the cardiovascular system, cleanses the respiratory system, increases strength and stamina, lowers serum cholesterol, relaxes the nervous system, stimulates pain-killing brain chemical activity, reduces stress and brings a sense of overall peace and wellbeing. As creatures born of nature, we are fundamentally designed to 'use it or lose it'! Yet the word 'exercise' never fails to conjure up an immediate mental resistance in most of us. While we still automatically think of exercise as routine physical exertion that is nearly impossible to fit into our stressful everyday lives, this need not be the case. Our understanding of the concept of healthy movement has come a long way since the days of regimented aerobics classes and sweaty gyms. Experts now agree that the best forms of exercise, those that contribute to a well-balanced, long and healthy life, are activities that take into account our physical, mental and spiritual needs. There is no better place to realize these health and fitness goals than outdoors, in nature. It often takes some soul-searching and trial and error to find the forms of exercise that suit us best. Some people like the same exercise activity, year in and year out, while others thrive on variety. The options for outdoor exercise are enormous — walking, jogging, hiking, climbing, cross-country skiing, biking and swimming are the most popular. All are excellent cardiovascular activities that are all the more enjoyable when undertaken in fresh air, with a constantly changing view for mental stimulation. If you are someone who enjoys structured classes and gym workouts, you'll find that interspersing them with outdoor exercise will enhance your athletic abilities and bring your perception of health and fitness into clearer focus. Even the most exercise-resistant have had their lives changed by simply going down to their local humane societies and adopting a dog. In addition to opening your heart to another being who will happily be a faithful companion for life, owning a dog makes exercise — even a short walk around the block — a certainty!

Indoor activities like yoga, stretching and dancing all take their inspiration from age-old exercise forms and will increase your health and longevity. Yoga in particular accomplishes many of the goals of living the natural lifestyle. More than an exercise, yoga is a constantly evolving, 6,000 year old philosophy which embraces the physical, mental, emotional and spiritual aspects of life. The Yogic 'salute to the sun' sequence is one of the most perfect exercises, which, if done regularly, effortlessly builds aerobic capacity, stretches and strengthens the muscles, improves balance, flexibility and co-ordination, enhances breathing and eliminates residual stress. There are many different branches of Yoga practice to choose from, each with its own particular emphasis. Other forms of mind/body exercise movement include Tai Chi, martial arts, Pilates and stretching. Try to incorporate your chosen exercise forms into your life on a regular basis. As you become aware of the enormous benefits to your health as you indulge in enjoyable exercise, you'll wonder how you ever managed without it.

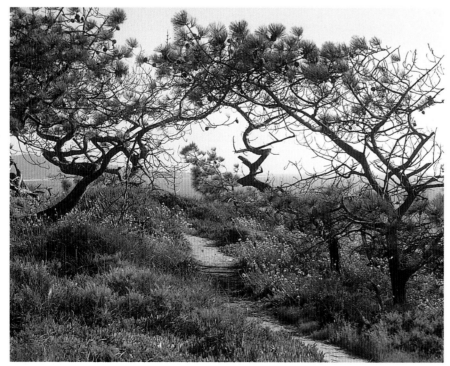

STRESS MANAGEMENT

Stress has been called the disease of modern civilization, and with good reason. Stress has been shown to depress and impair the functioning of the body's vital immune system, making it a major contributor to the progression of life-threatening illnesses. Even in its mildest forms, as presented in newspapers or on the nightly TV news, stress can undermine and derail the results of even the most conscientious person who is otherwise following all the guideposts of natural living. Stress manifests itself in many ways — anger, fear, self-criticism, negativity, panic, anxiety, depression, introversion, and physical and mental pain. The developing field of psycho-neuro-immunology has shown that external stressors initiate a complex set of responses within the body. Personal interactions with others, whether colleagues at work, family members, acquaintances or complete strangers, invariably create constant stresses in our lives. Relationship challenges, job insecurity, financial pressures, health concerns and the fast-paced and constant changes of modern life all breed internal fears, tensions and stress. Re-evaluating your work and home life in order to resolve existing stresses and learning to handle the events and mental patterns that create stress is of enormous importance if you plan on living a happy, long and fulfilling life. Fortunately, now there are many ways to handle stress.

Over the past few decades, many new therapies have evolved to help us learn to understand and cope with stress, nullifying its negative effects and even turning it to positive use in the form of manageable challenges. These modalities include

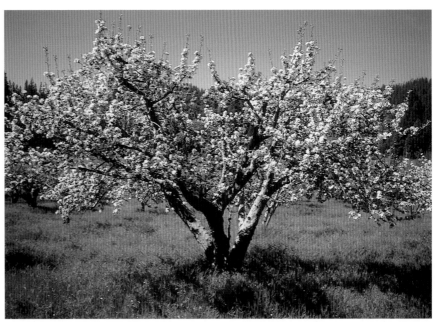

psychiatry, psychology, counseling, hypnotherapy, biofeedback, bodywork, meditation, creative visualization and imagery, among many others. There are many ways in which we can take control of stress ourselves, once we have learned to identify it. Breathing is the most immediate and effective way of negating stress. The moment you find yourself in an unpleasant, stressful situation, consciously take several deep breaths while keeping your mind fixed on a pleasant feeling or association that calms you. Since we usually respond to stress with either fear or anger, allow the immediate stressful feelings to wash over you, and keep breathing slowly and deeply until your anger or fear of the situation abates.

A natural partner to deep breathing is meditation, which can take many forms. In addition to traditional seated meditation, many people now find that they enjoy walking or moving meditation, especially outdoors, where they can enjoy the changing colors, aromas and moods

of the seasons. The trend towards 'mindfulness' or unhurried, conscious meditation while engaged in everyday pursuits is gaining enormous popularity. 'Mindfulness' teaches us to view ourselves as part of the natural world, savoring our connection with it in every detail. Inner reflection and a focused simplicity in thought and action help us to overcome the unending crises that stress attempts to impose on us. Creative visualization is another practice that has caught our collective imagination in our stressful times. Imagery and visualization techniques often encourage us to imagine ourselves in an ideal natural setting where we feel happy and secure, in order to effect positive changes in real life. The power of the mind to change and heal stressful situations cannot be underestimated. If stress is affecting your ability to achieve total health and wellbeing, seek out the natural stress management modalities that work for you, and customize them to become a healing part of your new balanced, natural life.

NATURE'S HEALING POWER AT HOME

A simpler life, one more attuned to the natural world, allows us to live in greater harmony with ourselves and others. Nowhere is this more important than in our homes, where we sleep, entertain, bathe, relax, and increasingly, work. Once you have established a healthy pattern of diet, exercise and stress management, your life will automatically become much calmer and clearer, and you will want to reflect this in your home environment. Your home is the most unique expression of the way you live, so keeping it clean and uncluttered will give you a sense of order and renewed creativity. When redecorating, find comfortable furniture that you can live with, and select natural materials and textures including wood, stone and glass. Select neutral, serene colors and natural textures in fabrics and drapes. Ensure that your home has sufficient ventilation and is enhanced by natural light and sunshine. Since so many of us now work at home, a cheerful and organized workspace is important, ideally one which lets in natural light and provides a pleasing outside view. Being able to look out and see restful natural scenery is very grounding and centering, so orient your home office with this in mind.

You may want to look into 'feng shui', the ancient Chinese art of design and placement, which ascribes 'chi' or life energy to objects and spaces. In feng shui, thoughtful planning of your home or office and the auspicious placement of objects within them will attract good energy and prosperity to you. Natural objects like indoor plants, flowers, mirrors, wind chimes, crystal gemstones, fountains,

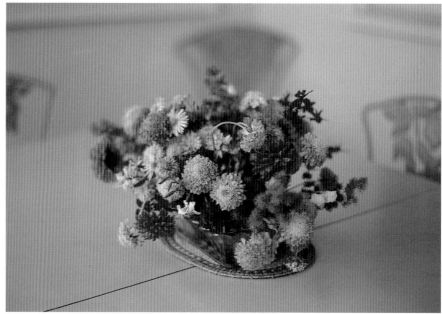

water and fish aquariums are believed to foster good 'chi' when they are positioned harmoniously. Photographs, personal treasures, mementos and symbolic objects that have meaning to you can be kept in a small area where you can see them frequently and be aware of their presence. Color, light and sound are integral to feng shui. Determine which colors you gravitate towards and bring them into your home in the form of plants and flowers, fabrics and artwork. Be sure that lighting in your home is soft and pleasing, and use candles whenever possible. Music is one of the most healing powers there is. Whatever your musical preference, listening to music provides balance, equilibrium and inspiration. Nature sounds — waterfalls, wind, rain, ocean surf and birdsong — are extremely relaxing and healing for many people. As much as possible, allow the sensory delights of nature to bring harmony and peace into every room in your home. If you can, use natural ventilation to connect your home to the larger 'room' of nature.

If you are fortunate enough to have a garden, you already know how relaxing and pleasurable it is to work in it and watch it change through the seasons. If not, see if you can become involved in a community garden or create a small potted garden on a rooftop or terrace. While you may feel that gardening is a new or unfamiliar venture, you will soon find the creativity and energy it inspires addictive. Even the smallest space can support living, growing things. Window boxes and terracotta pots on balconies yield a surprising amount of herbs, vegetables and colorful flowers. The healing power of flowers is undeniable, as anyone who has received them while in the hospital can testify. Try to have fresh flowers in your home as often as possible; their aroma, color and graceful beauty inspire and instill serenity in everyone. Surrounding yourself with natural, living things will remind you to stay in touch with yourself, keep you in harmony with nature, and will have great positive effects on your health, energy and wellbeing.

AROMATHERAPY FOR HEALTH AND WELL-BEING

Pure essential oils, being derived from naturally-grown plants, herbs and flowers, are potent healing substances that are considered to contain the life force and vitality of the plants themselves. The beauty of aromatherapy is that we are able to bring the positive, health-promoting qualities of these plant essences into our lives very easily. Pure essential oils have a variety of different effects on the mind and body. Some are stimulating and energizing, some are balancing and regulating, while others are deeply relaxing and calming. Their tiny molecules readily vaporize in the air and are detected as subtle, pleasing aromas when inhaled. Once inhaled or applied to the skin, essential oils are absorbed rapidly and exert their therapeutic effects on the body systems. The versatility of the oils is remarkable — they can be used directly in ceramic and electric diffusers, aroma-lamps and candles, as well as in baths, showers, footbaths and compresses. When added to oils and lotions, they transform a massage or body treatment, and can be custom-blended to meet every health and beauty need.

Have some fun with aromatherapy by selecting a favorite oil or two, and including them in daily 'rituals', for inhalation, bathing, skincare and relaxation. Peppermint, for instance, is a classic 'morning' oil with a fresh, clean invigorating aroma which is ideal for starting your day off right. Japanese researchers have even designed alarm clocks that wake you up with energizing aromas! Use drops of peppermint oil on a damp cloth in the shower or use a peppermint-infused gel. A drop of oil in water makes an excellent morning mouth rinse, and rubbing a little peppermint lotion around your sinuses and temples will clear your head and prepare you for the full day's work ahead. A personal diffuser at your desk using peppermint or another energizing oil will keep you alert and refreshed through your busy day. For the morning, select from

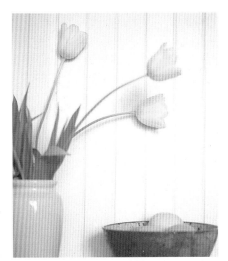

uplifting oils such as basil, bergamot, clary sage, eucalyptus, grapefruit, juniper berry, lemon, orange, peppermint, petitgrain, pine, rosemary, spearmint and verbena.

Once the day's work is done, you may feel the need to wind down and regroup before going home or preparing dinner. The late afternoon hours call for essential oils having balancing, regulating properties. These oils adjust your mood and metabolism gently before the relaxation of the evening sets in. Select a favorite oil or oil blend (known as a 'synergy', as two to three oils combined have a greater therapeutic value than the sum of their parts) from the range of balancing oils, which include cedarwood, chamomile, cypress, geranium, lavender, mandarin, melissa, palmarosa, rosewood and ylang-ylang. If you are going to be in an environment that would benefit from a little freshening, include eucalyptus, lemon, pine, sage, tea tree or thyme in your blend. Sniff any of these oils from a tissue as you head for home, or better still, use a car diffuser that is activated by the heat of the lighter in your vehicle. Once you arrive home, you will be feeling calm yet balanced, unaffected by rush-hour stress.

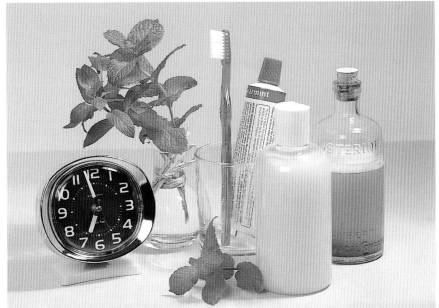

Home is your sanctuary, so here's where you can really unwind! The rich and exotic oils and absolutes of true aromatherapy love the evening hours! Absolutely nothing can beat the hedonistic joy of an evening bath with sensuous oils like neroli, ylang-ylang or sandalwood. Let everyone know that you are indulging in quiet time. Dispatch the kids to do their schoolwork or watch TV, turn down the volume on the phone, dim the lights and pour your bath, adding your own homemade aromatherapy bath formulas. Put on some relaxing music, light a few candles, and you're ready to rejuvenate body, mind and soul! You may want to select a particular oil, such as lavender, to make the focus of your bathing ritual. Light lavender aromatherapy candles, put mineral bath salts and some drops of lavender oil in the tub, and use lavender bodycare oil or lotion when you emerge from the fragrant water. Lie down and rest for a moment or two with an eye pillow filled with grains and lavender flowers to relax your eyes,

calm your mind and block out the outside world. A spritz of lavender mist and a drop of lavender essential oil on your pillow will ensure a good night's sleep.

If you're in the mood for romance, there are wonderful essential oils and absolutes to make your time with your partner special. With soft music in the air, fragrant candles burning, and sweet aromas surrounding you, the stage is set! Submerge yourself in bathwater made silky with milk bath, gels or oils, and pamper yourself and your partner with body oils and lotions using sensuous, exotic essences like rose, jasmine, neroli, sweet orange, sandalwood, patchouli, vanilla, benzoin, vetiver, frankincense or myrrh. Blend a sensual massage oil especially for your partner and indulge him or her in a long, relaxing full-body massage. Experiment with the essences and massage techniques to create different moods and fantasies. The oils will heighten your enjoyment and pleasure immensely.

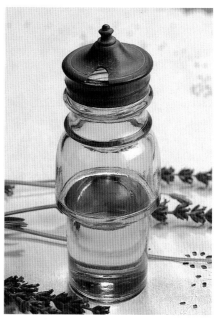

When the mood takes you, indulge in a 'spa day' at home using the different natural bodycare products you've made. Bathe, sip herb tea, do a yoga video, give yourself a facial, deep-condition your hair, treat your feet to reflexology, read a good book, and simply relax! Keep a diffuser or candle burning so you can benefit from inhaling the healing oils throughout your day. Try to fit aromatherapy massage into your life as often as possible. Massage using pure essential oils is the most important thing you can do to care for yourself, manage your stress and improve your physical and emotional health and wellbeing. Many bodywork professionals provide treatments in the privacy of your own home. You might also want to consider contacting a local massage school where students are putting in their hours towards accreditation, and arranging to receive regular aromatherapy massages in exchange for a reasonable fee. There are many creative ways you can receive and share the gifts that true aromatherapy will bring to your life.

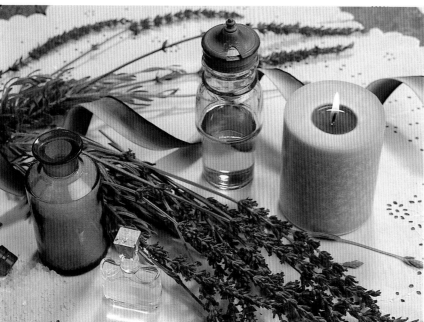

In conclusion, once you have experienced the benefits that true aromatherapy brings into your life, you will feel transformed. The stresses and pressures of daily living will seem much more manageable, and your energy, vitality and enthusiasm for life will improve greatly. You will be able to exert greater control over your physical and emotional health through the use of your own natural bodycare preparations, diet, exercise, stress management, relaxation techniques and natural healing methods. Lifestyle changes will be made with greater ease now that you have the tools and awareness. You'll have made the connection between good health and living the natural lifestyle. Here's wishing you a long, healthy and fulfilling life!

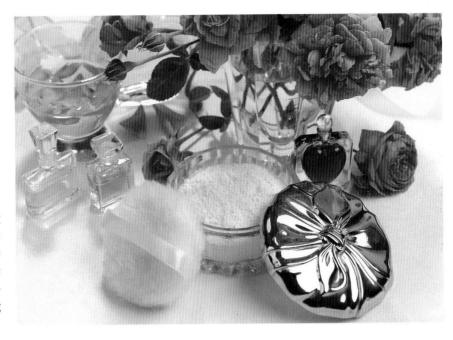

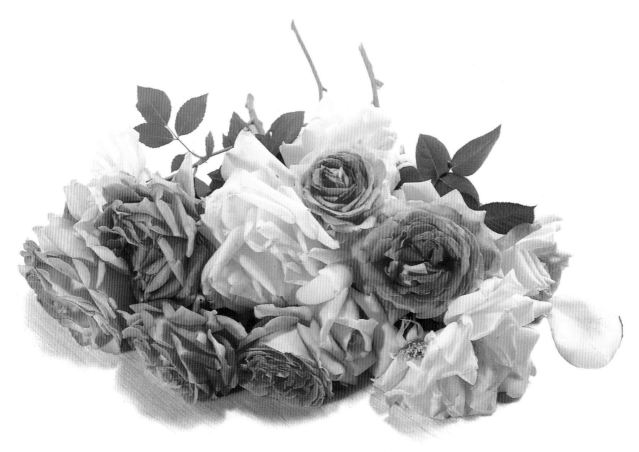

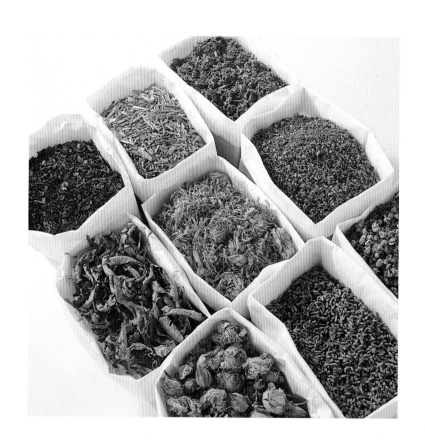

Dedication

This book is dedicated to my husband, Orville Recht,
whose confidence in me and my work has been a constant source of inspiration.

Acknowledgments

Special thanks to the following:

Treasures of Ojai, for their gracious loan of antiques and collectibles for photography
Carrol Gettko, publicist, for her loyal friendship and encouragement
Bryon and Jenni Frovarp of Frovarp Designs, for professional computer graphic layout
William B. Dewey, photographer and friend, for his inspired photographic work
Jane Kennedy at Palmetto, Laura and Aaron Reisfeld at Sabia Botanicals, Ron Robinson at Fred Segal Apothia,
Mr. and Mrs. Asahi and Andy Morishita, and our other progressive retailers and customers
All our friends, clients and visitors over the years: thanks for your support!
Liz Vernand, Dottie Briggs, Gina Garcia, Julianne Lee, Marcia Middendorf and Sandra Murillo at Essential Aromatics,
for minding the store, and
Charles G. Nurnberg, Executive Vice President of Sterling Publishing Co. Inc., for opening the door.

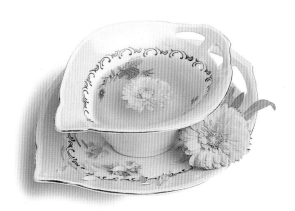

If you have questions, comments or need information on any of the special projects in this book, please call or write:
Essential Aromatics
205 North Signal Street
Ojai, CA 93023
(800) 211-1313

Index

Index to Recipes